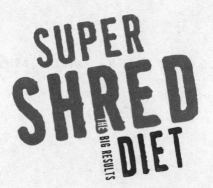

SUPER
SHRED
THE BIG RESULTS
DIET

ALSO BY IAN K. SMITH, M.D.

SHRED

The Truth About Men

Eat

Happy

The 4 Day Diet

Extreme Fat Smash Diet

The Fat Smash Diet

The Take-Control Diet

Dr. Ian Smith's Guide to Medical Websites

The Blackbird Papers: A Novel

SUPER SHRED

THE BIG RESULTS

DIET

4 WEEKS, 20 POUNDS, LOSE IT FASTER!

Ian K. Smith, M.D.

ST. MARTIN'S GRIFFIN NEW YORK

SUPER SHRED: THE BIG RESULTS DIET. Copyright © 2013 by
Ian K. Smith, M.D. All rights reserved. Printed in the United States
of America. For information, address St. Martin's Press,
175 Fifth Avenue, New York, N.Y. 10010.

www.stmartins.com

The Library of Congress has cataloged the hardcover edition as follows:

Smith, Ian, 1969–
    Super shred: the big results diet : 4 weeks 20 pounds lose it faster! /
Ian K. Smith.
      p. cm.
    Includes index.
    ISBN 978-1-250-04453-2 (hardcover)
    ISBN 978-1-4668-4291-5 (e-book)
    1. Reducing diets.   2. Weight loss.   I. Title.
    RM222.2.S62228 2013
    613.2'5—dc23

                                2013031020

ISBN 978-1-250-06120-1 (trade paperback)

St. Martin's Griffin books may be purchased for educational, business,
or promotional use. For information on bulk purchases, please
contact the Macmillan Corporate and Premium Sales Department at
1-800-221-7945, extension 5442, or write to
specialmarkets@macmillan.com.

First St. Martin's Griffin Edition: January 2015

10 9 8 7 6 5 4 3 2 1

I dedicate this work of labor to Damian Cherry,

Lisa Vines, Little Damian, Dante, and Omar.

The new crew at 62. Always in my heart,

forever in my love. Here's to you all!

Note to the Reader

This book is for informational purposes only. The author has endeavored to make sure it contains reliable and accurate information. However, research on diet and nutrition is evolving and subject to interpretation, and the conclusions presented here may differ from those found in other sources. As each individual's experience may vary, readers, especially those with existing health problems, should consult their physician or health-care professional before adopting any nutritional changes based on information contained in this book. Individual readers are solely responsible for their own health-care decisions, and the author and the publisher do not accept responsibility for any adverse effects individuals may claim to experience, whether directly or indirectly, based on information contained herein.

Contents

Acknowledgments

Whenever I see my name splashed across the front of a book for all to see, I always feel it's a shame that so many other names can't fit on the cover. The truth of the matter is that the stupendous effort and hard work that go into creating, processing, marketing, designing, selling, and publishing a book belong to a big team that largely goes unrecognized—until now. So, in no particular order but just out of recall: Elizabeth Beier, Michelle Richter, Steve Cohen, Sally Richardson, John Karle, Katie Bassell, Michael Storrings, Jeff Dodes, Lorraine Saullo, and John Cusack, and the entire St. Martin's sales team. I am so appreciative of your belief in me and my books and the countless hours you dedicated to making my vision a reality.

I want to give a special acknowledgment to my publisher, Matthew Shear. He was quite simply a prince of a man and always ready to roll up his sleeves to "publish the hell outta books." This is to you, Matthew. May your memory be a blessing. I will miss you tremendously.

Thanks to all of the SHREDDERs coast to coast who make up SHREDDER Nation and who have made me so proud and given me all of the feedback to make this program the best it can be. Your success is the fuel for my creative engine. Last but most important: Tristé, Dashiell, and Declan. I accomplish only because you make me strong and proud and inspire me to be better and happier. My love for you is endless. I hope I make you smile.

Introduction

Five years ago if you had asked me whether I would ever create a plan whose number one goal was to deliver very rapid weight loss, I would've looked at you like you had two heads. Along with many other dieting experts I have had a strong voice in the familiar chorus: "Slow, steady weight loss wins the day." But my e-mail inbox and Twitter feed weren't exactly listening to this song. Barraged by people who wanted to get the weight off fast without pills or surgery, I started exploring what was long considered impossible by many—rapid but *healthy* weight loss.

The success of my previous book, *SHRED: The Revolutionary Diet*, taught me a lot about the ability of well-meaning and determined people to actually lose more than a pound a week—the number always suggested as a goal by experts. The average result on SHRED in six weeks' time was 4 inches and two sizes. SHREDDERs across the nation started local SHREDDER support groups on Facebook, where they support one another, exchange recipes, offer advice, and even meet up to work out. Our national Facebook page, www.face book.com/ShredderNation, has become a place for tens of thousands of SHREDDERs to communicate, provide support, and hear the latest as it concerns weight loss and living a healthier life.

Despite the success and vast appeal of SHRED, the question of losing weight rapidly still came up. So I hunkered down and read through the research again and looked at some new, exciting concepts that took another approach to weight loss. I learned that for all of these years, the major reason why we had been advising people not to lose weight quickly was because they were typically using unhealthy methods to achieve their impressive goals. So what if I could create a program that could deliver these big results in a short period of time but did so in a healthy way that did not put the dieter in harm's way? Welcome to SUPER SHRED.

The plan is short, but because it demands that you be at your best, there can be times when you're tempted to eat an extra snack, increase the size of a meal, or skip a workout. When you feel like you're close to giving in to this temptation, write these words on a piece of paper and keep the paper with you so that you can read it whenever you start getting those feelings of doubt.

I have a big goal that I'm trying to reach in a short time.

I really want above everything else to see myself reach this goal.

I will do what it takes for just this short period of time to reach this goal.

I CAN and MUST and WILL stick to the plan for victory.

It's also helpful if you enlist a friend or some type of support system who can give you honest and immediate feedback when you feel like you're close to making a bad decision. Call, e-mail, or text your support, let them know what you're going through, and tell them that you need them to help you get through this moment. We all find inspiration in different places, sometimes in our children, a vision of what we see happening in the future, a smile we want to see on someone else's face when we succeed. Whatever inspiration you have used in the past to make it against the odds, employ that same inspiration during your tough moments over the next four weeks.

This program delivers because those who truly want these results are willing to do the work. No program that is healthy and reasonable can shave off the pounds if you are going to be sedentary and eat too much harmful food all day and not give it your best effort. Many might dream of this type of plan, but it simply doesn't exist. So I went to SHREDDER Nation on Facebook and Twitter and put what I thought was a solution to the test. The results were absolutely amazing. The average weight loss in just four weeks was 20 pounds. Some even said they would've had even better results had they given it a little more effort.

SUPER SHRED is not built for long-term use—for that you should go to the original SHRED. No, SUPER SHRED is specifically built for a quick hit or boost when you need to get that weight off quickly because there's an event you're going to attend or a special occasion that's approaching and you want to look and feel your best. It's also built for those who might've been told by their doctors that they are pre-diabetic and in danger of having the full-blown disease or that, for the first time in their life, they have high blood pressure. Not only will SUPER SHRED help you knock the pounds off; it will lower blood glucose levels, normalize your cholesterol, and reduce your blood pressure. SUPER SHRED is engineered to be that quick fix, the holy grail of dieters, an answer to your weight-related problems that won't jeopardize your health. Some parts of the program are tough, and they're meant to be. If you're asking your body to lose the same amount of weight in four weeks that it's taken you three years to gain, then you must be challenged and pushed. There's simply no way around it. Your body can do amazing things, but you have to be willing to get up and get busy. Sticking to this plan and believing in yourself as well as in SUPER SHRED's core philosophy and strategy will help you achieve what you once might've thought impossible.

SUPER SHRED hard, my friends!

Ian K. Smith, M.D.
January 2014

For free weight loss and other health tips,
follow Dr. Ian
on Twitter: @doctoriansmith;
on the Web: www.doctoriansmith.com;
on Facebook: www.facebook.com/ShredderNation.
To receive a free copy of his digital newsletter, sign up at
www.doctoriansmith.com.
To purchase SHRED POP popcorn
and SHRED BARs, visit www.shredlife.com.

[CHAPTER 1]

The SUPER SHRED Concept

For many years I have been asked by tens of thousands of people, "How can I lose weight quickly?" For as long as I can remember, my answer was consistent. "Losing weight too quickly can be dangerous. It's best to lose it slow and steady so that you can keep it off longer."

Given the relevant science, I always accepted the conventional wisdom of steady weight loss being more beneficial than rapid weight-loss strategies. But I still wanted to explore whether it was actually possible to lose weight quickly *and* in a safe manner. I finally concluded that the answer is yes, but only after taking a step back to first understand why weight-loss experts continuously caution against the rapid weight-loss approach.

Programs that have promised fast weight loss have for the most part been extreme and unhealthy. They propose either a severe restriction in calories; unregulated, non-FDA-approved supplements to help boost the metabolism; or eating plans that call for eliminating entire food categories. These programs have been successful for many, but the harm they can potentially do to the body can outweigh the potential benefits that one achieves with the weight loss. What good is losing 15 pounds quickly if it means you are damaging your kidneys? What good is losing 20 pounds if it means you are going to gain it all back and then some in three weeks once you stop whatever plan it is that you're following?

SUPER SHRED is specifically designed to be a short-term rapid-weight-loss plan. It is not meant for the long term. Instead, it is what I call *destination dieting.* You have a cruise to get ready for in two months? You have a reunion to attend in six weeks? You need to look your best at a wedding in four weeks? SUPER SHRED is your secret weapon to help deliver the results you want. But remember, secret weapons are best used only when the stakes are high. You have plenty of other weapons in your arsenal, but when you really need to deliver that knockout blow, then you call on your secret weapon. The element of surprise that is so critical on the battlefield is also critical in the weight-loss battle. If you overuse the same weapon, your enemy knows what to expect and can defend against it better, and eventually the weapon becomes less effective. Overusing SUPER SHRED can have the same impact on the effectiveness of the plan, which is why you should use it in short bursts.

The original plan, outlined in *SHRED: The Revolutionary Diet,* is meant to be the plan you can follow for the long term. It's a practical, inexpensive, straightforward program that delivers amazing results. In six weeks, the average person loses 4 inches and two sizes. People who have followed the original SHRED plan have mixed it up with SUPER SHRED to give themselves a boost. The results have been amazing, with the average weight loss each week being just over 5 pounds.

SUPER SHRED is a four-week program that is constructed in a way that will deliver the best results. There is flexibility built into the plan, but it's important to do your best to follow it as written. Our time to deliver is short, so that means there's little time to deviate and recover. This makes every day important, and it makes it necessary for you to plan, prepare, and execute as efficiently as possible. If you're going to do SUPER SHRED, make sure you have time to do it and that you're not trying to do it when you're distracted or not in control of your food environment. For best results, follow the program when you can give it all of the mental and physical attention it deserves and needs.

Weight loss in general is not easy. It requires lifestyle changes and breaking bad habits that have spun you and your scale out of control. It's easy to want the quick fix, but you have to be willing to put in the work that's necessary to achieve the results. SUPER SHRED is not a tough program, but it can be demanding, and it's purposely built this way. If your body is not challenged, then it will not transform. SUPER SHRED will push you, but it will not overwhelm you. You will get as much out of it as you put into it, so your expectations should match the level of intensity at which you choose to do the plan.

As with any weight-loss plan, the amount of weight people lose will vary. Our tests have shown that the average weight loss in four weeks is 20 pounds. But you have to understand the context of these results. Some people lost less, some people lost more. No two people lose weight in the same way or at the same pace. Some will lose pounds first, while others will lose inches first. Some lose them both at the same time. We are all made differently and respond differently to diets. Never compare yourself to someone else or you will set yourself up for disappointment. You are your own comparison and that's what you should be thinking as you begin SUPER

SHRED. Think about how *you* have lost weight in the past and then compare your results on SUPER SHRED with those experiences.

How much weight you lose in these four weeks will depend on a lot of variables. There are many medical conditions—for example, hypothyroidism—that can slow or impede weight loss. There are many classes of medications—for example, steroids or drugs to control blood pressure—that have a side effect of weight gain, and this means they can impair your ability to lose weight. It also matters how much weight you really need to lose and how close you are to your target weight. Someone who has only 20 pounds to lose is most likely not going to lose it as fast as someone who needs to lose 60 pounds. It's a generally recognized axiom of weight loss that the closer you are to your target weight, the more difficult it is to lose the weight. Don't take it personally. It's just the way our bodies work. What you need to understand is that the body becomes comfortable and doesn't want to release those last 15 or 20 pounds, so it puts up a fight not to let them go. This doesn't mean you can't lose them, but it does mean you have to be focused and determined and work hard to win.

There are many strategies at work in SUPER SHRED, but the three that are most critical are negative energy balance, calorie disruption, and sliding nutrient density. While each one alone can bring success when it comes to weight loss, I have merged all three into one program so that you can draw from the entire group and achieve maximal results.

Negative Energy Balance

Negative energy balance is an extremely important concept when it comes to weight loss and it's especially important in SUPER SHRED.

The concept is rather simple. Energy balance describes the relationship between the calories that are consumed through food and drink (energy in) and calories that the body uses throughout the day during all activities (energy out). This relationship determines whether one maintains weight, loses weight, or gains weight.

Negative energy balance means that the energy you consume is less than the energy you expend. When your body is in this state, it is looking for energy, because it's not getting enough in food and drinks. The body has three major sources of energy—carbohydrates, fats, and protein. Your body also tends to use those sources in that particular order. Fat is a great source of energy, which is why we need it to live. When we consume more energy than we actually burn off, the body stores this energy in our fat cells. When the body needs energy to perform activities such as exercising, putting away dishes, or eating, it will use the energy found in carbohydrates first, but this runs out pretty quickly. The body will then go into the fat cells to get the energy that it has been storing. Proteins are the last to be tapped.

SUPER SHRED puts your body in a state of negative energy balance so that you will go into your fat stores for the energy, thus reducing the amount of fat while at the same time losing pounds. Exercise is critical during this four-week program, because it will create the demand for energy and thus the need to burn fat to get this energy. The calories you consume each day have been particularly measured so that your body will achieve this state of negative energy balance. You won't need to count calories during the entire program, as I have done all of that for you, but you will need to pay attention to the instructions regarding sizing and portions of food and drinks.

Calorie Disruption

It is common knowledge by now that in order to lose weight, the calories coming in must be fewer than the calories going out. Emerging research, however, has added some new twists to this old truth. Scientists have been taking a closer look at important issues such as metabolism, calorie consumption, and fasting. As you can imagine with new concepts, not everyone is in agreement, but there is enough preliminary evidence to elicit serious interest from major research institutes.

Intermittent fasting is a concept in which one fasts on a given number of days. The basic strategy calls for alternating days where you eat "normally" with days in which your calorie consumption is not completely eliminated but severely restricted. For example, you might eat 2,500 calories five days in a row, then eat 700 calories a day for the next two days. These two days are called your fasting days. Some small studies have shown that this can be as effective as or more effective than counting calories every day to lose weight. But the research shows that there are more benefits than just what you record on the scale. Some of the evidence has shown that blood pressure is reduced, levels of sugars and fats in circulation are improved, and inflammation—an indicator of heart disease risk—can be limited.

Despite the need for larger and longer studies, intermittent fasting remains a potentially promising concept that could yield big weight-loss results. SUPER SHRED employs an aspect of intermittent fasting that I call calorie disruption. The reduction of calories is not as severe as you will find in typical intermittent-fasting regimens, but the daily calories are meticulously planned so that you do experience abrupt shifts in the amount you consume. This is represented particularly by the SUPER SHREDDER days. Each week there is a day in which the amount of calories you consume will be quite different from what you have consumed earlier in the week and what you will consume later in the week. It's very important during these days to stick to the plan and make sure you eat all of your snacks and meals that day. This is a day that you will be particularly challenged, but if you plan correctly and remember what this day represents, then you will be fine. Most important is the psychological aspect to the SUPER SHREDDER day. Having a positive attitude is critical. You must remember that it is only 24 hours, and you can do *anything* for 24 hours.

Beyond the SUPER SHREDDER day, your calories are on a roller coaster between meals and even between the non–SUPER SHREDDER days. Once again, you won't be counting calories, but the foods, beverages, and portion sizes I have selected will keep challenging your body with their variety and thus have an impact on your metabolism. The ability to alter your metabolism through food choices and to match this alteration with the exercise program can make a huge difference in the results that you eventually achieve.

In the original SHRED program, calories were altered from week to week, but SUPER SHRED has more dramatic alterations. The rises and dips and turns in this program constantly challenge you and make your body search for new stability. The trick, however, is that this stability is rarely if ever achieved, thus leading to a state of instability that consequently causes you to need more calories and effectively burn more fat.

Sliding Nutrient Density

Most people are omnivores, meaning they eat both plants and animals. Entire books have been written about whether a diet dominated by plants or meat is healthier. While meat in moderation and cooked in a healthy way can contribute important nutrients to your diet, a plant-based diet remains the healthiest eating style with regard to disease prevention, a longer life span, and weight loss.

Nutrient density is the quantity of nutrients you get for the number of calories contained in that food or beverage. The ideal situation is to get the most nutrients for the fewest calories. In other words, nutrient-dense foods give you the biggest nutritional bang for your calorie buck. SUPER SHRED works because it provides you with tremendous nutrient density and it does so by sliding the cuisine away from heavy meats, cream sauces, and carbohydrate-rich foods that provide only some nutrients but at the cost of a lot of calories. Instead, the ratio is changed in the SUPER SHRED plan so that you are loading up on healthy nutrients but minimizing the amount of calories you consume.

You can have vegetables, meat, and fish; however, the way the daily menus are constructed, the majority of your choices in the later part of each day will be plant-based instead of meat-based. In other words, this is an omnivore's diet with a lot of nutrient density, but it tilts toward the plant aspect, thus loading you up on all kinds of disease fighters such as antioxidants and fiber. This strategy also means that you will be reducing the number of calories you consume through the day, with your earlier meals typically being heavier than those that come later in the day. This is important, because as we become less active later in the day and have less time to burn off calories, we want to make sure the foods we consume also contain fewer calories.

Eating meat or fish is not mandatory in SUPER SHRED. Vegetarians of all types can have great success with this program. Simply make the necessary substitutions where you need to in the daily menus, and you will be completely fine.

SUPER SHRED Weeks

There are four weeks of SUPER SHRED, and each one can stand on its own. Each week, however, does weave into the larger plan, so the weeks work on a progressive strategy. Each week has a different theme and purpose. The four weeks symbolize what is happening during SUPER SHRED—losing weight F-A-S-T.

Foundation is the first week. Because we have only four weeks to attain the desired results, it's important to jump right in. This is the easiest of the weeks and it sets a good foundation for you to successfully complete the rest of the program. You will understand the importance of meal timing and preparation and how to pace yourself so that your exercise and eating are synchronized to give you the results you desire. Most people lose 5 pounds this week; some lose even more. Results do, however, vary and depend on a host of factors.

Accelerate is the second week, and it looks and feels different from Foundation week. This week is specifically designed to push you. Most people see a dramatic slowdown during the second week of any weight-loss program. To help you avoid such a plateau, this week is designed to help you accelerate through the natural slowdown. You might not lose as much weight as you did during the first week, but you will keep losing and avoid the second-week blues. The push in this week is critical, since at its completion you will be halfway through the program.

Shape is the third week of the program and carries this name because this is the week in which your body's metamorphosis really takes shape and you and others will start to notice a distinct difference. You will see changes in the shape of your body and the fit of your clothes, and the acknowledgment from others that you are losing weight becomes frequent and gratifying. This is absolutely the toughest week of the program. This is the week you will experience true calorie disruption. This week is specifically designed to be challenging but not overwhelming. You will get through these seven days, and after doing so, you will gain a greater confidence and respect for what you are actually capable of doing once you put your mind and body to it.

Tenacious is the fourth and last week of SUPER SHRED. It's not the easiest week of the plan, but it's not the most difficult, either. Coming after the highly challenging week 3, this week will seem practical and quite doable. This week is called Tenacious because it's important that you remain determined and stubborn to close out the program. Temptations must be resisted during this final stretch, and at this point you should be on top of your game. You know what it takes to make it through a week of SUPER SHRED, so now it's time to employ all that you have learned and developed in this last push toward your goal. Nothing can stop you when you're tenacious!

[CHAPTER 2]

How SUPER SHRED Works

SUPER SHRED **is a program designed to bring you fast results,** but in a healthy way. The plan is laid out in a very simple, easy-to-follow strategy. Each day you will have a detailed meal plan that you will follow. There will be some flexibility in the meal plan so that you can have choice in what you eat and drink. Timing is important for the plan to be most effective, so try your best to set a schedule and stick to the guidelines that are recommended for that week.

Each week is different, so pay attention to the eating instructions for that week as well as the schedule of meals. Sometimes you will have three snacks, sometimes only two. Some weeks you will have four meals, others only two. Each week is specifically designed so that no two are alike. This is why it's so important to pay attention to the week's layout at the beginning of each chapter.

Skipping meals is a big mistake, and it can be counterproductive on SUPER SHRED. If you are not hungry enough to eat all of the meal, then don't eat it all. Just eat some of it. But skipping it altogether is not the solution. Your body must grow accustomed to a regular eating schedule, as it is counting on those energy calories to nourish and fuel it so it can carry out the basic functions of life. Eat until you are satisfied, not stuffed. We all know what it feels like to be so stuffed you can barely get up from the table. It might've tasted great going down, but then it sits in your stomach and you don't even want to move. If you stuff yourself, you have overeaten, and that is exactly the opposite of what we're trying to accomplish with SUPER SHRED. This plan will help you improve your relationship to food and become more in tune with your body's true needs rather than what you think your body needs.

Substitutions

SUPER SHRED is a program that provides flexibility, which makes it accessible to almost anyone. Whether you suffer from a medical condition, have a food allergy, or have food preference restrictions, you can still follow this plan. While it's advised to make as few changes to the plan as possible, you can definitely make substitutions where necessary. Great care has gone into structuring this program so that you can achieve maximum results, so be aware that modifying it too much can also impact your chances of succeeding.

While I have tried to cover as many scenarios as possible, no one diet can take into account all the possibilities or questions that can arise. This is why old-fashioned common sense is important and needs to be employed when you are in doubt. If you become confused or find yourself unsure, err on the side of caution. Vegetables, for example, can always be substituted in the program. You can never go wrong by choosing them. But that also means cooking them properly. For example, fried green tomatoes, while quite tasty, are not a proper substitution while on this diet. The goal is to eat as cleanly as possible, so when you are faced with a choice, choose the item that's lower in calories, closer to how it exists in nature (less processed), and most abundant in nutrients such as vitamins, minerals, fiber, and protein. The idea is that you can take SUPER SHRED on the road with you, whether eating out at a restaurant, a friend's house, or on vacation. It's a portable program. Even in difficult food environments you should be able to find something that will work and hold you over until you have better choices available.

Exercise

I am quite aware that for many people, exercise is the word they do not want to hear. But in SUPER SHRED, it is a part of the program you will come to enjoy. Remember that you are asking your body to deliver some extremely impressive results in an extremely short period of time. To accomplish this, all strategies need to be in synch and operating at maximum capacity. Hands down, exercise is the best way to boost your metabolism and burn up the energy that your fat cells have been storing.

Each day a certain amount of time is recommended for your exercise. You are expected to do at least that amount of time. If you are motivated to do even more, that's great. Go ahead and do it. You will have certain days marked as rest days. If you still want to do something on those days, that's fine also. The more work you put in with your exercise program, the better the results you will achieve.

The *SHRED 27 Burn* DVD is a 27-minute workout that has been specifically designed with the SHREDDER in mind. Find out more about it at www.doctoriansmith.com. Many people are surprised at how short this workout is compared to the hour or more they've been told to do by trainers and others. This high-intensity interval training program is great for burning calories, improving your endurance, and increasing your energy levels. Once you get the DVD, you can follow it as instructed; if you want to do another workout on some days, that is fine also. Variety in the type of workout you do is strongly encouraged and will keep your metabolism boosted while preventing you from getting bored with the program.

The SUPER SHRED exercise requirements typically center on cardio exercises. This does not mean that you can't do resistance training—free weights or bands. You can add resistance training in your second week of the program. You shouldn't need more than 25 to 35 minutes to do a good resistance-training program. Try to do this three times a week. Remember, however, that we are not trying to build bulky muscle, but rather nice lean muscle. That means lifting light weights for a high number of repetitions. So, for example, if you were to do arm curls with 5-pound dumbbells, you should be lifting the weights for fifteen repetitions per set. You should do three sets for that particular exercise maneuver. If you can't do this, then that means the weight is too heavy for our purpose. It might help to get a few sessions with a trainer at a local gym so that you understand the correct form, body posture, and safety while lifting weights. Resistance training in addition to the cardio exercises that you will be doing can go a long way in boosting your metabolism and helping to burn the fat faster by creating the ever-important negative energy balance.

Maintenance

SUPER SHRED is not meant to be a long-term program. I can't emphasize this enough. SUPER SHRED is your secret weapon when you want to lose weight quickly but in a healthy manner. I have designed this program so that you can employ it on an as-needed basis, not as a way to eat for the rest of your life. Remember, *destination dieting*. Once you have done SUPER SHRED and you want to maintain your loss or even lose a little more, then you should go back to the original SHRED diet plan.

SUPER SHRED has been constructed to fit perfectly with the original SHRED. The daily menus and the flexibility in the program have been designed to make your transition to SHRED quite seamless. Given the great results you find with SUPER SHRED, you might be inclined to go through another four-week cycle. Doing consecutive cycles is fine, but I suggest that you don't do more than two in a row. You should at least do the six-week SHRED cycle before you attempt another SUPER SHRED cycle. It's important that your body not grow accustomed to eating and exercising in the same manner, and this is why cycling on and off SUPER SHRED and using the original SHRED as your life plan can not only bring the best results but provide you with the best opportunity to maintain them.

CHAPTER 3

Week I: Foundation

Welcome to your first week of **SUPER SHRED**. This is going to be an exciting journey, but before you go any further, you must agree that during the next four weeks you will absolutely give your best effort to stick to the plan, minimize excuses, and keep pushing yourself even when you're discouraged or things seem difficult. The first week is critical, as it sets up your chances for success for the remaining three weeks. This is why it is called your Foundation week. You will build upon this week, and it's important to create your good habits now so they will carry you through the rest of the program.

You are asking a lot of your body as far as achieving great results in a short period of time, so you have to give this your best. The more work you put in, the better the results you will get out. Because time is limited, you really need to hit the ground running. Each day you stick to the program is one day you get closer to your goal. Each day you overeat, skip more than one meal, or eat food that's not on the daily menu is considered a slip, and it takes you backward, away from your goal. If you slip when you are less than halfway through the week (days 1 to 3), go back to the beginning of the week. If you slip on any of days 5 to 7, just go back one day and do it again. If you slip on day 4, do day 4 again. Minor slips, such as having one extra small snack or eating your meal 30 minutes later than scheduled, do not necessitate your starting over. No one is perfect and you're not expected to be. But at this point you will know if you had a major slip or just a minor slip. Not being honest about it only affects you and your results, so you are cheating no one but yourself and the results you will achieve by the end of the week.

The table below shows a sample schedule for timing your meals and snacks. Timing is essential, as it distributes your calories in a way that keeps your fat-burning metabolism maximized and keeps your insulin hormone levels as stable as possible. Erratic hormone levels can cause weight gain, so the meal spacing structured in this program seeks to avoid hormone spikes as much as possible. Please note that this is only a sample. All of us get up and go to sleep at different times, so you have to set your schedule accordingly. If you keep in mind that the meals are 3 to 4 hours apart and the snacks are 1½ hours after the meal that precedes it, then you will be fine.

7:30 A.M.	8:30 A.M.	10:00 A.M.	11:30 A.M.	12:30 P.M.	4:30 P.M.	7:30 P.M.
Awake	Meal 1	Snack 1	Snack 2	Meal 2	Meal 3	Meal 4

Make sure you read all of the guidelines before beginning the plan, and since they are so short and convenient, feel free to circle back at any time during the week to check on things that you might have a question about. If your question still isn't answered, err on the side of caution by eating less or not eating a food that might not be allowed on the plan. Remember, we don't have a lot of time to lose this weight, so making good decisions is critical. It's okay to set the bar high, but it's not okay to make choices that are going to sabotage your chances of success. Regardless of what that number reads on the scale at the end of this week, if you gave it your best shot, that is the best you can do and that's the most you can ask of yourself. You still have three more weeks to produce results, so don't get upset and hang your head. We all lose weight at different speeds and in different places. Don't compare yourself to anyone else. Believe! Work really hard! Smile and have lots of fun, especially during the tough times!

SUPER SHRED Week I Grocery List

This is a list that takes into consideration the different combinations of food and beverage items offered to you this week. Because the program has a lot of flexibility and choices, no one list can be constructed for everyone. In the list below you will find food and beverage opportunities. You can make the choices that fit your preferences and purchase accordingly. Note that there are some items that you *must* have. You should be sure to buy them so that you will have them on hand when the program calls for them. If you are a vegetarian, you don't need to eat the meat meals. Make appropriate substitutions, but be mindful of calorie counts.

FRUIT
- **Must:** 2 lemons
- **Must:** 6 additional servings of fruit. This can be a combination of berries and other fruits.
- **Serving size:** 1 piece of fruit = 1 serving; ½ cup of berries = 1 serving

BREAKFAST OPTIONS

- **Must:** 6 breakfast meals. Choose your combination from this list.

3 cups oatmeal (1 cup cooked = 1 meal)

1 cup Cream of Wheat (1 cup cooked = 1 meal)

4 cups sugar-free or low-sugar (under 5 grams) cereal: for example, Kashi 7 Whole Grain Puffs, Cheerios, Fiber One (1 cup = 1 meal)

2 eggs (2 eggs = 1 meal)

1 loaf of bread

2 pancakes, preferably whole-grain (size of a CD)

1 strip of bacon (turkey or pork)

1 low-fat or fat-free 6-ounce yogurt

1 grilled cheese sandwich made with 2 slices of regular cheese on 2 pieces of 100 percent whole-wheat or whole-grain bread

BEVERAGES

- **Must:** 6 cups green tea or hibiscus tea.
- **Must:** 32 additional drink options for the week. Water is not included; you may have as much as you want. Choose your combinations from the list below. Then purchase your choices for the week.

27 cups of fresh juice

14 cups of coffee

7 twelve-ounce cans of diet soda

21 cups of low-fat, reduced-fat, or fat-free milk or unsweetened soy or almond milk

21 cups of unsweetened iced tea

20 cups of lemonade

2 cups of flavored water

SALADS

- **Must:** 4 large green garden salads, 1 small green garden salad
- **Optional:** You will have other opportunities to have salads. Those opportunities are listed below. You should choose which of these you want, then purchase accordingly.

3 medium green garden salads

1 large green garden salad

1 small green garden salad with turkey sandwich

VEGETABLES

- **Must:** 12 servings
- **Optional:** 3 servings. You will have other vegetable opportunities. If you choose them, purchase accordingly.
- **Serving size:** 1 serving is approximately the size of your fist; for a tomato, 1 serving is a medium tomato.

MEAT AND FISH

- **Must:** 4 servings. Choose from the list below. But note the maximum number of servings you may have for each option.
- **Optional:** 1 serving
- **Serving size:** 1 serving = 5 ounces, cooked, approximately the size of a deck and a half of playing cards.
- Your maximum number of servings for this week if you choose all of the optional servings is 5 servings. Make your choices

from the list below, mixing them up. Remember, you must have at least 4 servings. For example, you can choose to have 3 pieces of lean beef, 1 piece of chicken, and 1 piece of fish. But you can't have 5 pieces of lean beef. You can have 3 total.

3 pieces of lean beef

3 pieces of chicken

5 pieces of fish

4 pieces of turkey

SNACKS

- Choose fourteen snacks for the entire week, such as nuts, popsicles, chocolate-covered strawberries, and other items listed in chapter 7. Remember, snacks are encouraged, but optional.

7 SHRED BARs or other snack items 150 calories or less

7 bags SHRED POP popcorn or other snack items 100 calories or less

SOUPS, SMOOTHIES, PROTEIN SHAKES

- **Must:** 1 cup of soup
- **Must:** 12 additional servings from the items listed below. Each item must be 200 calories or less, with no added sugar. Choose the combination that you desire and purchase accordingly.

9 cups of low-salt soup (less than 480 milligrams sodium)

9 fruit smoothies

8 protein shakes

OPTIONAL MEAL CHOICES

- Throughout the week you will have the opportunity to have the meals listed below. Choose which of them you want, then purchase accordingly. You can choose all or none of them.

1 cup of pasta

2 slices of small cheese pizza (no larger than 5 inches across the crust and 5 inches long)

1 serving of lasagna, with or without meat (4 inches × 3 inches × 1 inch)

1 veggie burger (3 inches in diameter, ½ inch thick)

EXTRAS

- These are things you might want to have on hand during the week, so stock up on them.

Diced vegetables

1 dessert of 100 calories or less

1 stick of butter

1 small jar of jelly

Sugar packets (helps with portion control)

Half-and-half

1½ tablespoons of syrup

1 tablespoon of grated cheese

Extra milk for cereal

Ground beef for pasta

Marinara sauce for pasta

1 slice of cheese for turkey sandwich

Mustard

Mayo

Tomato

Lettuce

SUPER SHRED Week I Guidelines

• Weigh yourself in the morning the day you start the program
and make sure you record it. You will weigh yourself only once a
week, so even if you are tempted, stay off the scale. Your body naturally fluctuates a couple of pounds from day to day. Measuring
yourself every day could give you an inaccurate weight and unnecessarily stress you and lead you to believe you're not succeeding.
Your next weigh-in will be exactly a week from your initial weigh-in.
Make sure you weigh yourself in the same manner each time: if you
weighed in wearing certain clothes or no clothes at all, make sure
you do the same the second time around and as close to the same
time of the day. Make sure you use the same scale both times, as
different scales can be off by several pounds, thus destroying the
accuracy of your measure.

• Do not skip meals. Even if you're not hungry, just have something during the allotted time. You can always grab a piece of fruit
or something small during your mealtime. Also, you don't have to
eat all of the meal. You can eat just some of it. If you're not hungry,
don't stuff yourself. Just eat a little. The key is to eat at regularly
scheduled times so that your body grows accustomed to these eating times. Each week will change, so it's important to quickly adapt
to the week that you're in and its related schedule. During the

course of the week you should never go more than 4 hours without eating something. Your meals should be 3 to 4 hours apart. Your snacks should fall about 1½ hours after meals. If you miss a meal or snack, you can't save it and eat it later or combine them. Once that time has passed, move on and hit your next mark.

• All of your shakes and smoothies this week must be 200 calories or less. If you follow the recipes in the back of the book, they will fit this description. If you buy them from a store, be sure of the calorie count. Also, be mindful of the serving sizes of the drinks. If the recipe makes more than one serving, be sure you drink only one at that time. If the store-bought product contains more than 1 serving, just drink the equivalent of 1 serving and refrigerate the rest for next time.

• Snacks are optional, but highly recommended. The SHRED BARs and SHRED POP popcorn are suggested for many of your snacks, as they are specifically made with all the nutritional guidelines in mind. However, you may have other snacks as long as they fall under the proper calorie count. There is plenty of diversity when it comes to snacks, so take advantage of it.

• Soups are an option, including store-bought soups. But make sure you look at the sodium content: no more than 480 milligrams *per serving.* Be mindful of the serving size. For the purpose of this plan, 1 serving is equivalent to 1 cup, whether you eat store-bought soup or make it fresh. You may have 1 saltine cracker with your soup.

• Consume 1 cup of water before *every* meal.

• You are allowed 2 cups of coffee each day, 1 cup at breakfast and the other whenever you like. Stay away from all those fancy coffee preparations—lattes, Frappuccinos, coffees that pile on the calories. A tablespoon of sugar and a little half-and-half or milk won't hurt, but don't go overboard. Keep your coffee clean.

• Canned and frozen fruits and vegetables are allowed. Please be aware of added ingredients. Make sure they are either packed in water or labeled "no sugar added." The key is to have food in its most natural state with the least amount of processing. Make sure you check the sodium levels, as they can be quite high: try to keep the amount to 480 milligrams of salt for any serving of food.

• While fresh-squeezed juice is definitely preferred, you can drink store-bought juice. Just make sure it says "not from concentrate" and "no sugar added." If you're a diabetic or have trouble regulating your blood sugar, choose a different beverage option, such as water, milk, or tea.

• The program doesn't spell out alcohol choices in the beverage section, but you are allowed to have a total of 3 alcoholic drinks for the week: 2 mixed drinks *or* 3 light beers *or* 3 glasses of wine *or* a combination of these drinks. Note serving sizes: 1 beer = 12 fluid ounces; 1 serving of wine = 5 fluid ounces (a little more than half a cup); a mixed drink has about 1½ fluid ounces of hard liquor. Also, you can't have them all in one day, so there's no saving them up for a big hit during the weekend. Liquid calories are stealthy and count just as much as food calories! And they definitely cause weight gain!

• You are allowed 1 diet soda per day if you desire. Regular soda is not recommended.

• Do not eat your last meal within 90 minutes of going to sleep. If because of circumstances you're eating late and know you're going right to bed, then consume half the meal.

• Spices are unlimited, so enjoy. Salt is not a spice. You are allowed to add no more than ½ teaspoon of salt to your food each day.

• If you are a vegetarian or diabetic or need to avoid certain foods owing to other medical conditions, it is completely acceptable to make substitutions. But make smart substitutions and be mindful of the portion sizes.

• Serving sizes: A 5-ounce serving of fish or meat, cooked, is typically the size of a deck and a half of playing cards. A serving of vegetables is typically the size of an adult's fist. A serving size of hot cereal is 1 cup of *cooked* cereal.

- You may have ½ pat of butter (about ½ teaspoon) with hot cereal.
- You may have 1 teaspoon of sugar (white or brown) with cereal, or ½ teaspoon of honey with hot cereal.
- If you must switch days or meals within a day for scheduling reasons, try to do so as infrequently as possible.
- If you need to rearrange your exercise regimen for scheduling reasons, it is permissible to do so.

SUPER SHRED WEEK 1, DAY 1

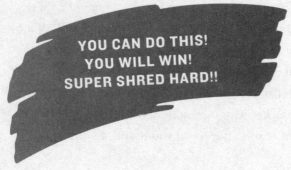

YOU CAN DO THIS!
YOU WILL WIN!
SUPER SHRED HARD!!

MEAL I

- 1 piece of fruit. Choose from the following, though you may choose others: pear, apple, ½ cup of raspberries or strawberries or blueberries or blackberries, banana, ½ cup sliced melon, ½ grapefruit, ½ cup of cherries.
- Choose one of the following:

1 cup of oatmeal

1 cup of sugar-free cereal with low-fat, reduced-fat, or fat-free milk or unsweetened soy or almond milk

2 egg whites or 1 egg-white omelet with diced veggies prepared with cooking spray or a little oil or butter

Optional: 1 piece of 100 percent whole-grain or whole-wheat toast (½ pat butter or ½ teaspoon jelly)

BEVERAGES

- **Must:** 1 cup of green tea or 1 cup of hibiscus tea (dash of sugar acceptable)
- **Must:** 1 cup of water
- **Optional:** 1 cup of fresh juice or 1 cup of coffee (no more than 1 packet of sugar, 1 tablespoon of milk or half-and-half)

SNACK 1

- 1 SHRED BAR *or* 1 cup of grape tomatoes *or* 1 medium sliced red bell pepper with ¼ cup guacamole *or* another item 150 calories or less

SNACK 2

- 1 SHRED POP popcorn *or* 2 medium kiwis *or* 1 cup of blueberries with 1 tablespoon of whipped cream *or* another item 100 calories or less

MEAL 2

- Choose one of the following. Your choice must not exceed 200 calories; no sugar added.

1 protein shake

1 fruit smoothie

1 cup of soup (no potatoes, no heavy cream). Good choices are chicken noodle, vegetable, lentil, chickpea, split pea, black bean, tomato basil, minestrone. Always be careful of sodium content!

BEVERAGES

- Choose one of the following:

Unlimited plain water (flat or fizzy)

1 cup of lemonade

1 cup of unsweetened iced tea

1 cup of juice (not from concentrate)

12-ounce can of diet soda (no more than 1 per day)

1 cup of low-fat, reduced-fat, or fat-free milk or unsweetened soy or almond milk

MEAL 3

- 1 large green garden salad (4 cups of greens). You may include a few olives, shredded carrots, and ½ sliced tomato or 5 grape tomatoes. Only 3 tablespoons of fat-free dressing, no bacon bits, no croutons.

BEVERAGES

- Choose one of the following. Try to choose a different beverage from the one you chose in meal 2.

Unlimited plain water (flat or fizzy)

1 cup of lemonade

1 cup of unsweetened iced tea

1 cup of juice (not from concentrate)

12-ounce can of diet soda (no more than 1 per day)

1 cup of low-fat, reduced-fat, or fat-free milk or unsweetened soy or almond milk

MEAL 4

- 1 cup of water before eating
- 2 servings of vegetables
- Choose one of the following:

5-ounce piece of lean beef (grilled or broiled)

5-ounce piece of chicken (baked or grilled, not fried, no skin)

5-ounce piece of fish (baked or grilled, not fried)

5-ounce piece of turkey (not fried, no skin)

BEVERAGES

- Choose one of the following. Try to choose a different beverage from the ones you chose in meals 2 and 3.

Unlimited plain water (flat or fizzy)

1 cup of lemonade

1 cup of unsweetened iced tea

1 cup of juice (not from concentrate)

12-ounce can of diet soda (no more than 1 per day)

1 cup of low-fat, reduced-fat, or fat-free milk or unsweetened soy or almond milk

Exercise

- **Amount of exercise today:** minimum 40 minutes. If you want to do more, all the better! Work as hard as you can! The key is to avoid doing steady-state exercise such as walking on the treadmill at the same speed and same incline for a period of time. Instead, try to vary your speed, your incline, the distances you cover. The goal here is to do high-intensity interval training.

- **Option 1:** Do the *SHRED 27 Burn* workout DVD.
- **Option 2:** Choose two of the cardiovascular exercises below, for a total of 40 minutes of exercise.

Walking/running outside or on treadmill

Jogging outside

Elliptical machine

Stationary or mobile bicycle

Swimming laps

Stair climber

200 jump rope revolutions

20-minute treadmill intervals

Zumba or other cardio dance workout

SUPER SHRED WEEK 1, DAY 2

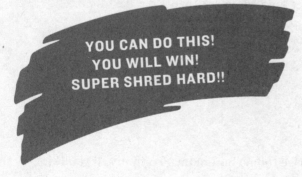

YOU CAN DO THIS!
YOU WILL WIN!
SUPER SHRED HARD!!

MEAL I

- 1 piece of fruit or ½ cup of berries
- Choose one of the following:

2 pancakes (diameter of a CD), preferably whole-grain, and 1 strip of bacon (turkey or pork) with 1½ tablespoons of syrup

2 egg whites scrambled with diced vegetables if desired (a little butter or cooking spray allowed)

1 cup of sugar-free cereal with low-fat, reduced-fat, or fat-free milk or unsweetened soy or almond milk.

BEVERAGES

- **Must:** 1 cup of green tea or 1 cup of hibiscus tea (a dash of sugar is allowed)
- **Must:** 1 cup of water with fresh lemon juice squeezed in (use half a lemon)
- **Optional:** 1 cup of coffee (no more than 1 packet of sugar, 1 tablespoon of milk or half-and-half)

SNACK 1

- 1 SHRED BAR *or* ½ blueberry muffin *or* 1½ cups of fruit salad *or* another item 150 calories or less

SNACK 2

- 1 SHRED POP popcorn *or* ⅓ cup of wasabi peas *or* 10 baby carrots *or* another item 100 calories or less

MEAL 2

- Choose one of the following. Your choice must not exceed 200 calories; no sugar added.

1 protein shake

1 fruit smoothie

1 cup of soup (no potatoes, no heavy cream). Good choices are chicken noodle, vegetable, lentil, chickpea, split pea, black bean, tomato basil, minestrone. Always be careful of sodium content!

BEVERAGES

- Choose one of the following:

Unlimited plain water (flat or fizzy)

1 cup of lemonade

1 cup of unsweetened iced tea

12-ounce can of diet soda (no more than 1 per day)

1 cup of low-fat, reduced-fat, or fat-free milk or unsweetened soy or almond milk

MEAL 3

- 1 large salad. You may have some sliced grilled chicken on the salad and any veggies; 4 tablespoons of fat-free or low-cal dressing; no bacon bits, no croutons.

BEVERAGES

- Choose one of the following. Try to choose a different beverage from the one you chose in meal 2.

Unlimited plain water (flat or fizzy)

1 cup of lemonade

1 cup of unsweetened iced tea

1 cup of juice (not from concentrate)

12-ounce can of diet soda (no more than 1 per day)

1 cup of low-fat, reduced-fat, or fat-free milk or unsweetened soy or almond milk

MEAL 4

- Start with 1 cup of water before eating your first bite.
- 2 servings of vegetables
- Choose one of the following:

1 cup of pasta with marinara sauce (but *no* cream sauces)

1 large green garden salad (4 cups of greens). You may include a few olives, shredded carrots, a few slices of beets, onions, and ½ sliced tomato or 5 grape tomatoes. Only 3 tablespoons of fat-free dressing, no bacon bits, no croutons.

6 ounces of fish (baked or grilled, not fried)

BEVERAGES

- Choose one of the following. Try to choose a different beverage from the ones you chose in meals 2 and 3.

Unlimited plain water (flat or fizzy)

1 cup of lemonade

1 cup of unsweetened iced tea

1 cup of juice (not from concentrate)

12-ounce can of diet soda (no more than 1 per day)

1 cup of low-fat, reduced-fat, or fat-free milk or unsweetened soy or almond milk

Exercise

- **Amount of exercise today:** minimum 35 minutes. If you want to do more, all the better! Work as hard as you can! The key is to avoid doing steady-state exercise such as walking on the treadmill at the same speed and same incline for a period of time. Instead, try to vary your speed, your incline, the distances you cover. The goal here is to do high-intensity interval training.
- **Option 1:** Do the *SHRED 27 Burn* workout DVD.

- **Option 2:** Choose two of the cardiovascular exercises below, for a total of 35 minutes of exercise.

Walking/running outside or on treadmill

Jogging outside

Elliptical machine

Stationary or mobile bicycle

Swimming laps

Stair climber

200 jump rope revolutions

20-minute treadmill intervals

Zumba or other cardio dance workout

SUPER SHRED WEEK 1, DAY 3

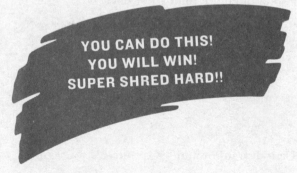

YOU CAN DO THIS!
YOU WILL WIN!
SUPER SHRED HARD!!

MEAL I

- 1 piece of fruit or ½ cup of berries
- Choose one of the following:

1 six-ounce container of low-fat or fat-free yogurt

2 pieces of whole-grain toast (½ pat butter or ½ teaspoon jelly)

1 scrambled egg (diced veggies optional, 1 tablespoon of grated cheese allowed, little butter or cooking spray allowed)

1 cup of sugar-free cereal with low-fat, reduced-fat, or fat-free milk or unsweetened soy or milk

BEVERAGES
- **Must:** 1 cup of green tea or 1 cup of hibiscus tea (dash of sugar allowed)
- **Must:** 1 cup of water
- **Optional:** 1 cup of fresh juice or 1 cup of coffee (no more than 1 packet of sugar, 1 tablespoon of milk or half-and-half)

SNACK 1
- 1 SHRED BAR *or* 16 cashews *or* ½ cup of roasted chickpeas *or* 1 large apple sliced and sprinkled with cinnamon *or* another item 150 calories or less

SNACK 2
- 1 SHRED POP popcorn *or* 1 baked medium tomato with 2 teaspoons of parmesan cheese *or* 2 stalks of celery *or* another item 100 calories or less

MEAL 2
- Choose one of the following:

1 turkey sandwich on 100 percent whole-grain or whole-wheat bread with a teaspoon of mustard or mayo, a slice of tomato, lettuce, and 1 slice of cheese. With your sandwich you may have a piece of fruit or a small green garden salad (2 cups of greens that can include a couple of olives, shredded carrots, a couple of small

slices of tomato; only 1 tablespoon of fat-free dressing; no bacon bits, no croutons).

1 cup of soup (no potatoes, no heavy cream). Good choices are chicken noodle, vegetable, lentil, chickpea, split pea, black bean, tomato basil, minestrone. Always be careful of sodium content!

3 servings of vegetables (a serving is typically the size of your fist)

1 protein shake not to exceed 200 calories; no sugar added

1 medium green garden salad (3 cups of greens). You may include a few olives, shredded carrots, a few slices of beets, onions, and ½ sliced tomato or 5 grape tomatoes. Only 2 tablespoons of fat-free dressing, no bacon bits, no croutons.

BEVERAGES

- Choose one of the following:

Unlimited plain water (flat or fizzy)

1 cup of lemonade

1 cup of unsweetened iced tea

1 cup of juice (not from concentrate)

12-ounce can of diet soda (no more than 1 per day)

1 cup of low-fat, reduced-fat, or fat-free milk or unsweetened soy or almond milk

MEAL 3

- 2 servings of vegetables
- Choose one of the following:

5-ounce piece of lean beef (grilled or broiled)

5-ounce piece of chicken (no skin, not fried)

5-ounce piece of fish (baked or grilled, not fried)

5-ounce piece of turkey (no skin, not fried)

BEVERAGES

- Choose one of the following. Try to choose a different beverage from the one you chose in meal 2.

Unlimited plain water (flat or fizzy)

1 cup of lemonade

1 cup of unsweetened iced tea

1 cup of juice (not from concentrate)

12-ounce can of diet soda (no more than 1 per day)

1 cup of low-fat, reduced-fat, or fat-free milk or unsweetened soy or almond milk

MEAL 4

- Start with 1 cup of water before taking your first bite.
- 1 cup of soup (no potatoes, no heavy cream). Good choices are chicken noodle, vegetable, lentil, chickpea, split pea, black bean, tomato basil, minestrone. Always be careful of sodium content!
- 1 serving of vegetables
- Dessert 100 calories or less, such as a scoop of fat-free ice cream, raspberry bar, or citrus-infused strawberries

BEVERAGES

- Choose one of the following. Try to choose a different beverage from the ones you chose in meals 2 and 3.

Unlimited plain water (flat or fizzy)

1 cup of lemonade

1 cup of unsweetened iced tea

1 cup of juice (not from concentrate)

12-ounce can of diet soda (no more than 1 per day)

1 cup of low-fat, reduced-fat, or fat-free milk or unsweetened soy or almond milk

Exercise

- **Amount of exercise today:** minimum 40 minutes. If you want to do more, all the better! Work as hard as you can! The key is to avoid doing steady-state exercise such as walking on the treadmill at the same speed and same incline for a period of time. Instead, try to vary your speed, your incline, the distances you cover. The goal here is to do high-intensity interval training.
- **Option 1:** Do the *SHRED 27 Burn* workout DVD.
- **Option 2:** Choose two of the cardiovascular exercises below, for a total of 40 minutes of exercise.

Walking/running outside or on treadmill

Jogging outside

Elliptical machine

Stationary or mobile bicycle

Swimming laps

Stair climber

200 jump rope revolutions

20-minute treadmill intervals

Zumba or other cardio dance workout

SUPER SHRED WEEK 1, DAY 4
SUPER SHREDDER DAY

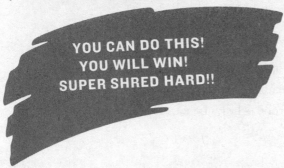

YOU CAN DO THIS!
YOU WILL WIN!
SUPER SHRED HARD!!

MEAL I

- **Must:** 1 cup of green tea or 1 cup of hibiscus tea (a dash of sugar is allowed)
- Choose one from the following. Your choice must not exceed 200 calories; no sugar added.

1 fruit smoothie

1 veggie or fruit juice (not from concentrate)

Optional: 1 cup of fresh juice or 1 cup of coffee (no more than 1 packet of sugar, 1 tablespoon of milk or half-and-half)

SNACK I

- 1 SHRED BAR *or* 1½ cups of frozen grapes *or* 1 slice of Swiss cheese with 8 olives *or* another item 150 calories or less

SNACK 2

- 1 SHRED POP popcorn *or* 1 thin rice cake with 1 tablespoon of peanut butter *or* ½ cup raisin bran *or* another item 100 calories or less

MEAL 2

- Choose one of the following. Your choice must not exceed 200 calories; no sugar added.

1 fruit smoothie

1 cup of soup (no potatoes, no heavy cream). Good choices are chicken noodle, vegetable, lentil, chickpea, split pea, black bean, tomato basil, minestrone. Always be careful of sodium content!

BEVERAGES

- Choose one of the following:

Unlimited plain water (flat or fizzy)

1 cup of unsweetened iced tea

1 cup of juice (not from concentrate)

12-ounce can of diet soda (no more than 1 per day)

1 cup of low-fat, reduced-fat, or fat-free milk or unsweetened soy or almond milk

MEAL 3

- Choose one of the following. Your choice must not exceed 200 calories; no sugar added.

1 protein shake

1 fruit smoothie

1 cup of soup (no potatoes, no heavy cream). Good choices are chicken noodle, vegetable, lentil, chickpea, split pea, black bean, tomato basil, minestrone. Always be careful of sodium content!

BEVERAGES

- Choose one of the following. Try to choose a different beverage from the one you chose in meal 2.

Unlimited plain water (flat or fizzy)

1 cup of lemonade

1 cup of unsweetened iced tea

12-ounce can of diet soda (no more than 1 per day)

1 cup of low-fat, reduced-fat, or fat-free milk or unsweetened soy or almond milk

MEAL 4

- Start with 1 cup of water before eating.
- Choose one of the following. Your choice must not exceed 200 calories; no sugar added.

1 protein shake

1 fruit smoothie

1 cup of soup (no potatoes, no heavy cream). Good choices are chicken noodle, vegetable, lentil, chickpea, split pea, black bean, tomato basil, minestrone. Always be careful of sodium content!

BEVERAGES

- Choose one of the following. Try to choose a different beverage from the ones you chose in meals 2 and 3.

Unlimited plain water (flat or fizzy)

1 cup of lemonade

1 cup of unsweetened iced tea

12-ounce can of diet soda (no more than 1 per day)

1 cup of low-fat, reduced-fat, or fat-free milk or unsweetened soy or almond milk

Exercise

- Rest Day! This is a rest day, especially if you are aching and your muscles need recovery. But if you feel up to it and you decide to do some exercise on your own, that is completely allowed. Thirty minutes of cardio training will always serve you well, so feel free to get in some extra work. Each exercise session will move you closer to your goal!

SUPER SHRED WEEK 1, DAY 5

YOU CAN DO THIS!
YOU WILL WIN!
SUPER SHRED HARD!!

MEAL I
- 1 piece of fruit. Choose from the following, though you may choose others: pear, apple, ½ cup of raspberries or strawberries or blueberries or blackberries, ½ grapefruit, ½ cup of cherries.
- Choose one of the following:

1 cup of oatmeal

1 cup of Cream of Wheat

1 cup of sugar-free cereal with low-fat, reduced-fat, or fat-free milk or unsweetened soy or almond milk

2 scrambled egg whites or 1 egg-white omelet with diced veggies (little butter or cooking spray allowed)

Optional: 1 piece of 100 percent whole-grain or whole-wheat toast (½ pat butter or ½ teaspoon jelly)

BEVERAGES

- **Must:** 1 cup of water (hot or cold) with fresh lemon juice squeezed in (use half a lemon)
- **Optional:** 1 cup of coffee (no more than 1 packet of sugar, 1 tablespoon of milk or half-and-half)
- **Optional:** 1 cup of fresh juice (not from concentrate)

SNACK 1

- 1 SHRED BAR *or* 6 dried figs *or* 1 medium pear and 1 cup of low-fat or fat-free milk *or* another item 150 calories or less

SNACK 2

- 1 SHRED POP popcorn *or* 3 teaspoons of natural peanut butter *or* 2 cups of watermelon chunks *or* another item 100 calories or less

MEAL 2

- Choose one of the following:

1 medium green garden salad (3 cups of greens). You may include a few olives, shredded carrots, a couple of slices of beets, onions,

and ½ sliced tomato or 5 grape tomatoes. Only 3 tablespoons of fat-free dressing, no bacon bits, no croutons.

1 fruit smoothie 200 calories or less; no sugar added

1 cup of soup 200 calories or less (no potatoes, no heavy cream). Good choices are chicken noodle, vegetable, lentil, chickpea, split pea, black bean, tomato basil, minestrone. Always be careful of sodium content!

BEVERAGES

- Choose one of the following:

Unlimited plain water (flat or fizzy)

1 cup of lemonade

1 cup of unsweetened iced tea

1 cup of juice (not from concentrate)

12-ounce can of diet soda (no more than 1 per day)

1 cup of low-fat, reduced-fat, or fat-free milk or unsweetened soy or almond milk

MEAL 3

- 1 large green garden salad (4 cups of greens). You may include a few olives, shredded carrots, a few slices of beets, onions, and ½ sliced tomato or 5 grape tomatoes. Only 3 tablespoons of fat-free dressing, no bacon bits, no croutons.

BEVERAGES

- Choose one of the following. Try to choose a different beverage from the one you chose in meal 2.

Unlimited plain water (flat or fizzy)

1 cup of lemonade

1 cup of unsweetened iced tea

1 cup of juice (not from concentrate)

12-ounce can of diet soda (no more than 1 per day)

1 cup of low-fat, reduced-fat, or fat-free milk or unsweetened soy or almond milk

MEAL 4

- Start with 1 cup of water before eating.
- 2 servings of vegetables
- Choose from the following:

5 ounces of fish (baked or grilled, not fried)

5 ounces of chicken (baked or grilled, not fried, no skin)

BEVERAGES

- Choose one of the following. Try to choose a different beverage from the ones you chose in meals 2 and 3.

Unlimited plain water (flat or fizzy)

1 cup of lemonade

1 cup of unsweetened iced tea

12-ounce can of diet soda (no more than 1 per day)

1 cup of low-fat, reduced-fat, or fat-free milk or unsweetened soy or almond milk

Exercise

- **Amount of exercise today:** minimum 45 minutes. If you want to do more, all the better! Work as hard as you can and go for it! The key is to avoid doing steady state exercise, which means, for example, walking on the treadmill at the same speed and same incline for a period of time. Instead, try varying all of the parameters. Vary your speed, vary your incline, vary the distances you cover. The goal here is to do high-intensity interval training.
- **Option 1:** Do the *SHRED 27 Burn* workout DVD.
- **Option 2:** Choose two of the cardiovascular exercises below, for a total of 45 minutes of exercise.

Walking/running outside or on treadmill

Jogging outside

Elliptical machine

Stationary or mobile bicycle

Swimming laps

Stair climber

200 jump rope revolutions

20-minute treadmill intervals

Zumba or other cardio dance workout

SUPER SHRED WEEK 1, DAY 6

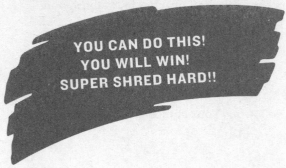

YOU CAN DO THIS!
YOU WILL WIN!
SUPER SHRED HARD!!

MEAL I

- 1 piece of fruit. Choose from the following, though you may choose others: pear, apple, ½ cup of raspberries or strawberries or blueberries or blackberries, ½ grapefruit, ½ cup of cherries.
- Choose one of the following. Your choice must not exceed 200 calories; no sugar added.

1 fruit smoothie

1 cup of sugar-free cereal with low-fat, reduced-fat, or fat-free milk or unsweetened soy or almond milk

BEVERAGES

- **Must:** 1 cup of green tea or 1 cup of hibiscus tea (dash of sugar allowed)
- **Optional:** 1 cup of fresh juice

SNACK I

- 1 SHRED BAR *or* 10 walnut halves and 1 sliced kiwi *or* 4 small deli turkey slices *or* another item 150 calories or less

SNACK 2

- 1 SHRED POP popcorn *or* 2 small peaches *or* 2 tablespoons of pumpkin seeds *or* another item 100 calories or less

MEAL 2

- Choose one of the following. Your choice must not exceed 200 calories; no sugar added.

1 protein shake

1 fruit smoothie

1 cup of soup (no potatoes, no heavy cream). Good choices are chicken noodle, vegetable, lentil, chickpea, split pea, black bean, tomato basil, minestrone. Always be careful of sodium content!

BEVERAGES

- Choose one of the following:

Unlimited plain water (flat or fizzy)

1 cup of lemonade

1 cup of unsweetened iced tea

1 cup of juice (not from concentrate)

12-ounce can of diet soda (no more than 1 per day)

1 cup of low-fat, reduced-fat, or fat-free milk or unsweetened soy or almond milk

MEAL 3

- 1 serving of vegetables
- Choose one of the following:

2 slices of cheese pizza (no larger than 5 inches across the crust and 5 inches long

1 serving of lasagna (with or without meat), 4 inches × 3 inches × 1 inch

1 veggie burger (3 inches in diameter, ½ inch thick)

1 medium green garden salad (3 cups of greens). You may include a few olives, shredded carrots, a few slices of beets, onions, and ½ sliced tomato or 5 grape tomatoes. Only 3 tablespoons of fat-free dressing, no bacon bits, no croutons.

BEVERAGES

- Choose one of the following. Try to choose a different beverage from the one you chose in meal 2.

Unlimited plain water (flat or fizzy)

1 cup of lemonade

1 cup of unsweetened iced tea

1 cup of juice (not from concentrate)

12-ounce can of diet soda (no more than 1 per day)

1 cup of low-fat, reduced-fat, or fat-free milk or unsweetened soy or almond milk

MEAL 4

- Start with 1 cup of water before eating.
- 1 small green garden salad (2 cups of greens). You may include a couple of olives, shredded carrots, a couple of small slices of tomato. Only 1 tablespoon of fat-free dressing, no bacon bits or croutons.
- Choose one of the following. Your choice must not exceed 200 calories; no sugar added.

1 protein shake

1 cup of soup (no potatoes, no heavy cream). Good choices are chicken noodle, vegetable, lentil, chickpea, split pea, black bean, tomato basil, minestrone. Always be careful of sodium content!

BEVERAGES

- Choose one of the following. Try to choose a different beverage from the ones you chose in meals 2 and 3.

Unlimited plain water (flat or fizzy)

1 cup of lemonade

1 cup of unsweetened iced tea

1 cup of juice (not from concentrate)

12-ounce can of diet soda (no more than 1 per day)

1 cup of low-fat, reduced-fat, or fat-free milk or unsweetened soy or almond milk

Exercise

- **Amount of exercise today:** minimum 40 minutes. Today you are going to do two exercise sessions. Do one session before 1 P.M. Do your other session after 4 P.M. Each session must be at least 20 minutes. If you want to do more, all the better, but at least 20 minutes per session! Work as hard as you can! The key is to avoid doing steady-state exercise such as walking on the treadmill at the same speed and same incline for a period of time. Instead, try to vary your speed, your incline, the distances you cover. The goal here is to do high-intensity interval training.

- **Option 1:** Do the entire *SHRED 27 Burn* workout in one session and half the workout in the other session. You can decide whether to do the full or the half session first.
- **Option 2:** Choose two of the cardiovascular exercises below, for a total of 40 minutes of exercise.

Walking/running outside or on treadmill

Jogging outside

Elliptical machine

Stationary or mobile bicycle

Swimming laps

Stair climber

200 jump rope revolutions

20-minute treadmill intervals

Zumba or other cardio dance workout

SUPER SHRED WEEK 1, DAY 7

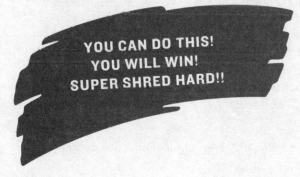

YOU CAN DO THIS!
YOU WILL WIN!
SUPER SHRED HARD!!

MEAL 1

- 1 piece of fruit. Choose from the following, though you can choose others: pear, apple, ½ cup of raspberries or strawberries or blueberries or blackberries, ½ grapefruit, ½ cup of cherries.

- Choose one of the following:

1 grilled cheese sandwich made with 2 slices of regular cheese on 2 pieces of 100 percent whole-wheat or whole-grain bread (little butter or cooking spray allowed)

1 cup of oatmeal

BEVERAGES

- **Must:** 1 cup of green tea *or* 1 cup of hibiscus tea *or* 1 cup of low-fat, reduced-fat, or fat-free milk or unsweetened soy or almond milk
- **Optional:** 1 cup of water
- **Optional:** 1 cup of fresh juice or 1 cup of coffee (no more than 1 packet of sugar, 1 tablespoon of milk or half-and-half)

SNACK I

- 1 SHRED BAR *or* 1 medium mango *or* 16 saltine crackers *or* another item 150 calories or less

SNACK 2

- 1 SHRED POP popcorn *or* 2 tablespoons poppy seeds *or* 6 oysters *or* another item 100 calories or less

MEAL 2

- Choose one of the following. Your choice must not exceed 200 calories; no sugar added.

1 protein shake

1 fruit smoothie

1 cup of soup (no potatoes, no heavy cream). Good choices are chicken noodle, vegetable, lentil, chickpea, split pea, black bean, tomato basil, minestrone. Always be careful of sodium content!

BEVERAGES

- Choose one of the following:

Unlimited plain water (flat or fizzy)

1 cup of lemonade

1 cup of flavored water

1 cup of unsweetened iced tea

1 cup of juice (not from concentrate)

12-ounce can of diet soda (no more than 1 per day)

1 cup of low-fat, reduced-fat, or fat-free milk or unsweetened soy or almond milk

MEAL 3

- 1 large green garden salad (4 cups of greens). You may include a few olives, shredded carrots, and ½ sliced tomato or 5 grape tomatoes. Only 3 tablespoons of fat-free dressing, no bacon bits, no croutons.

BEVERAGES

- Choose one of the following. Try to choose a different beverage from the one you chose in meal 2.

Unlimited plain water (flat or fizzy)

1 cup of lemonade

1 cup of unsweetened iced tea

1 cup of juice (not from concentrate)

12-ounce can of diet soda (no more than 1 per day)

1 cup of low-fat, reduced-fat, or fat-free milk or unsweetened soy or almond milk

MEAL 4

- Start with 1 cup of water before eating.
- 2 servings of veggies
- Choose one of the following:

5-ounce piece of chicken (no skin, not fried)

5-ounce piece of fish (baked or grilled, not fried)

5-ounce piece of turkey (no skin, not fried)

BEVERAGES

- Choose one of the following. Try to choose a different beverage from the ones you chose in meals 2 and 3.

Unlimited plain water (flat or fizzy)

1 cup of flavored water

1 cup of lemonade

1 cup of unsweetened iced tea

1 cup of juice (not from concentrate)

12-ounce can of diet soda (no more than 1 per day)

1 cup of low-fat, reduced-fat, or fat-free milk or unsweetened soy or almond milk

Exercise

- Rest Day! This is a rest day, especially if you are aching and your muscles need recovery. But if you feel up to it and you decide to do some exercise on your own, that is completely allowed. Thirty minutes of cardio training will always serve you well, so feel free to get in some extra work. Each exercise session will move you closer to your goal!

[CHAPTER 4]

Week 2: Accelerate

Congrats on making it to the second week of your **SUPER** SHRED journey. The fact that you have arrived here is success in and of itself. Regardless of what the number on the scale might read, if you gave it your best to stick to the plan the first week, then you have achieved. Success is not just how much weight you've lost, but includes other important aspects such as changing bad habits, improving your relationship with food and exercise, increasing energy, losing inches, and having a new attitude about what you can accomplish. Weight loss is very important, but it's only part of the bigger picture of overall wellness.

This is your second week of FAST results, and it is time to accelerate. Four weeks is not a long time, so our work must be immediate and diligent. This is the week we kick it up. In almost all diet plans, most people lose a significant amount of weight the first week, but the rate of loss slows down during the second week. But this doesn't have to be your experience with SUPER SHRED. To combat this natural tendency to slow down, you will have to fight it, remaining strict on meal portions and timing as well as completing the exercise program with vigor. The meals and snacks come in a different order this week, so pay close attention. Also, it's time to turn up the exercise. Push yourself to do more than just the minimum. The more you can put into this week, the more you will get out of it. Every day when you wake up and every night when you go to sleep, visualize the changes you are making and the transformation of your body. See yourself thinner and more sculpted. See that number on the scale decreasing with each week as you run toward your goal.

This week's schedule is different than last week's. You will now have three meals instead of four, but you will still have two snacks. Here is what a sample schedule might look like for someone who gets up at 7:30. Note that this is only a sample and you should build a schedule that works for your sleep-wake cycle and work-activity schedule. But be mindful of the basic guidelines. Waiting time between meal and snack should be 1½ hours, except the last snack, which can be eaten more than 1½ hours after the meal. The waiting time between meals this week is 3 to 4½ hours.

7:30 A.M.	8:30 A.M.	10:00 A.M.	12:30 P.M.	5:00 P.M.	8:00 P.M.
Awake	Meal 1	Snack 1	Meal 2	Meal 3	Snack 2

Make sure you read the guidelines that follow the grocery list. A lot of your questions will be answered if you take a few minutes to go through them instead of jumping right into the meal plan. Use the guidelines throughout the week to help you make the right choices. Substitutions are allowed, of course, but make them wisely.

SUPER SHRED Week 2 Grocery List

This is a list that takes into consideration the different combinations of food and beverage items offered to you this week. Because the program has a lot of flexibility and choices, no one list can be constructed for everyone. In the list below you will find food and beverage opportunities. You can make the choices that fit your preferences and purchase accordingly. Note that there are some items that you *must* have. You should be sure to buy them so that you will have them on hand when the program calls for them. If you are a vegetarian, you don't need to eat the meat meals. Make appropriate substitutions, but be mindful of calorie counts.

FRUIT
- **Must:** 1 lemon
- **Must:** 6 additional servings of fruit. This can be a combination of fruits such as berries, apples, bananas, pineapple, etc.
- **Optional:** small amount of fresh fruit to be added to low-fat yogurt
- **Serving size:** 1 piece of fruit = 1 serving; ½ cup of berries = 1 serving

BREAKFAST OPTIONS
- **Must:** 4 breakfast meals. Choose your combination from this list.

2 cups of oatmeal (1 cup cooked = 1 meal)

1 cup of Cream of Wheat or farina (1 cup cooked = 1 meal; instant is allowed)

4 cups of sugar-free or low-sugar (under 5 grams) dry cereal (1 cup = 1 meal)

2 eggs or ½ cup Egg Beaters (2 eggs = 1 meal)

1 loaf of bread

1 pancake the size of a CD

1 strip of bacon (turkey or pork)

3 six-ounce containers of low-fat plain yogurt

1 grilled cheese sandwich made with 2 slices of regular cheese on
2 pieces of 100 percent whole-grain or whole-wheat bread

1 cup of grits (1 cup cooked = 1 meal; instant is allowed)

BEVERAGES
- **Must:** 1 cup green tea or hibiscus tea
- **Must:** 21 drink options for the week. Water is not included;
  you may have as much as you want. Choose your combinations
  from the list below. Then purchase your choices for the week.

17 cups of fresh juice

7 cups of coffee

14 twelve-ounce cans of diet soda

14 cups of low-fat, reduced-fat, or fat-free milk or unsweetened
soy or almond milk

14 cups of unsweetened iced tea

14 cups of lemonade

14 cups of flavored water

SALADS
- **Must:** 2 large green garden salads, 1 small green garden salad
- **Optional:** You will have other opportunities to have salads.
  Those opportunities are listed below. You should choose
  which of these you want, then purchase accordingly.

1 large green garden salad

1 small green garden salad

VEGETABLES

- **Must:** 6 servings
- **Optional:** 4 servings. You will have other vegetable opportunities. If you choose them, purchase accordingly.
- **Serving size:** 1 serving is approximately the size of your fist.

MEAT AND FISH

- **Must:** 2 servings. Choose from the list below. But note the maximum number of servings you may have for each option.
- **Optional:** 3 servings
- **Serving size:** 1 serving = 5 ounces, cooked; approximately the size of a deck and a half of playing cards.
- Your maximum number of servings for this week if you choose all of the optional servings is 5 servings. Make your choices from the list below, mixing them up. Remember, you must have at least 3 servings.

2 chicken strips or prepared chicken fingers

1 cup of chicken stir fry

2 chicken sandwiches

2½-ounce piece of chicken

6 jumbo shrimp

3 five-ounce pieces of fish

1 five-ounce turkey burger

1 five-ounce piece of turkey

2 turkey sandwiches

1 four-ounce turkey burger

1 four-ounce hamburger

1 four-ounce veggie burger

1 five-ounce piece of lean country ham

SNACKS

- Choose fourteen snacks for the entire week, such as nuts, popsicles, chocolate-covered strawberries, and other items listed in chapter 7.

7 SHRED BARs or other snack items 150 calories or less

7 bags SHRED POP popcorn or other snack items 100 calories or less

SOUPS, SMOOTHIES, PROTEIN SHAKES

- **Must:** 4 cups of soup
- **Must:** 11 additional servings from the items listed below. Each item must be 200 calories or less, with no added sugar. Choose the combination that you desire and purchase accordingly.

3 cups low-salt soup (less than 480 milligrams sodium)

5 fruit smoothies

5 protein shakes

OPTIONAL MEAL CHOICES

- Throughout the week you will have the opportunity to have the meals listed below. Choose which of them you want, then purchase accordingly. You can choose all or none of them.

1 cup of pasta

1½ cups of brown rice

1 cup of beans, chickpeas, or lentils

EXTRAS

- These are things you might want to have on hand during Accelerate week.

Cheese for grilled cheese and other sandwiches

Extra milk for cereal and coffee

Salad toppings

Fat-free dressing for salad

2 tablespoons of cocktail sauce for shrimp

Sugar packets (helps with portion control)

Half-and-half

Mustard

Mayo

Tomato

Bun for burger

SUPER SHRED Week 2 Guidelines

- Weigh yourself in the morning the day you start the second week and make sure you record it. You will continue to weigh yourself only once a week, so even if you are tempted, stay off the scale. Your body naturally fluctuates a couple of pounds from day to day. Measuring yourself every day could give you an inaccurate weight and unnecessarily stress you and lead you to believe you're not succeeding. Your weigh-in will be exactly a week from this weigh-in. Make sure you weigh yourself in the same manner each time: if you weighed in wearing certain clothes or no clothes at all, make sure you do the same the next time around and as close to the same time of the day. Make sure you use the same scale each time, as different scales can be off by several pounds, thus destroying the accuracy of your measure.

• Do not skip meals. Even if you're not hungry, just have something during the allotted time. You can always grab a piece of fruit or something small during your mealtime. Also, you don't have to eat all of the meal. You can eat just some of it. If you're not hungry, don't stuff yourself. Just eat a little. The key is to eat at regularly scheduled times so that your body grows accustomed to these eating times. Each week will change, so it's important to quickly adapt to the week that you're in and its related schedule. During the course of the week you should never go more than 4 hours without eating something. Your meals should be 3 to 4 hours apart. Your snacks should fall about 1½ hours after meals. If you miss a meal or snack, you can't save it and eat it later or combine them. Once that time has passed, move on and hit your next mark.

• All of your shakes and smoothies this week must be 200 calories or less, with no sugar added. If you follow the recipes in the back of the book, they will fit this description. If you buy them from a store, be sure of the calorie count. Also, be mindful of the serving sizes of the drinks. If the recipe makes more than one serving, be sure you drink only one at a time. If the store-bought product contains more than 1 serving, just drink the equivalent of 1 serving and refrigerate the rest for next time.

• Snacks are optional, but highly recommended. The SHRED BARs and SHRED POP popcorn are suggested for many of your snacks as they are specifically made with all of the nutritional guidelines in mind. However, you may have other snacks as long as they fall under the proper calorie count.

• Soups are an option, including store-bought soups. But make sure you look at the sodium content: no more than 480 milligrams *per serving*. Be mindful of the serving size. For the purpose of this plan, 1 serving is equivalent to 1 cup, whether you eat store-bought soup or make it fresh. You may have 1 saltine cracker with your soup.

• Consume 1 cup of water before *every* meal.

• You are allowed 2 cups of coffee each day, 1 cup at breakfast. Stay away from all those fancy coffee preparations—lattes, Frappuccinos, coffees that pile on the calories. A tablespoon of sugar and a little half-and-half or milk won't hurt, but don't go overboard.

• Canned and frozen fruits and vegetables are allowed. Please be aware of added ingredients. Make sure they are either packed in water or labeled "no sugar added." The key is to have food in its most natural state with the least amount of processing. Make sure you check the sodium levels, as they can be quite high: try to keep the amount to 480 milligrams of salt for any serving of food.

• While fresh-squeezed juice is definitely preferred, you can drink store-bought juice. Just make sure it says "not from concentrate" and "no sugar added." If you're a diabetic or have trouble regulating your blood sugar, choose a different beverage option, such as water, milk, or tea.

• The program doesn't spell out alcohol choices in the beverage section, but you are allowed to have a total of 3 alcoholic drinks for the week: 2 mixed drinks *or* 3 light beers *or* 3 glasses of wine *or* a combination of these drinks. Note serving sizes: 1 beer = 12 fluid ounces; 1 serving of wine = 5 fluid ounces (a little more than half a cup); a mixed drink has about 1½ fluid ounces of hard liquor. Also, you can't have them all in one day, so there's no saving them up for a big hit during the weekend. Liquid calories are stealthy and count just as much as food calories! And they definitely cause weight gain!

- You are allowed 1 diet soda per day if you desire. Regular soda is not recommended.

- Do not eat your last meal within 90 minutes of going to sleep. If because of circumstances you're eating late and know you're going right to bed, then consume half the meal.

- Spices are unlimited, so enjoy. Salt is not a spice. You are allowed to add no more than ½ teaspoon of salt to your food each day.

- If you are a vegetarian or diabetic or need to avoid certain foods owing to other medical conditions, it is completely acceptable to make substitutions. But make smart substitutions and be mindful of the portion sizes.

- Serving sizes: A 5-ounce serving of fish or meat after being cooked is typically the size of a deck and a half of playing cards. A serving of vegetables is typically the size of an adult's fist. A serving size of hot cereal is 1 cup of *cooked* cereal.

- You may have ½ pat of butter (about ½ teaspoon) with hot cereal.

- You may have 1 teaspoon of sugar (white or brown) or ½ teaspoon of honey with hot or cold cereals.

- If you must switch days or meals within a day for scheduling reasons, try to do so as infrequently as possible.

- If you need to rearrange your exercise regimen for scheduling reasons, it is permissible to do so.

SUPER SHRED WEEK 2, DAY 1

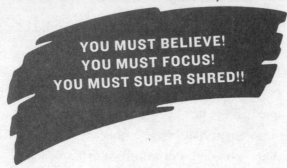

YOU MUST BELIEVE!
YOU MUST FOCUS!
YOU MUST SUPER SHRED!!

MEAL I

- 1 piece of fruit or ½ cup of berries.
- Choose one of the following:

1 cup of oatmeal

1 cup of Cream of Wheat or farina

1 cup of sugar-free cereal with low-fat, reduced-fat, or fat-free milk or unsweetened soy or almond milk

BEVERAGES

- **Must:** 1 cup of fresh juice (not from concentrate) or 1 cup of low-fat, reduced-fat, or fat-free milk, or unsweetened soy or almond milk
- **Optional:** 1 cup of coffee (no more than 1 packet of sugar, 1 tablespoon of milk or half-and-half)

SNACK I

- 1 SHRED BAR *or* 2 Fudgsicles *or* 1 small baked potato topped with salsa *or* any other item 150 calories or less

MEAL 2

- Choose one of the following. Your choice must not exceed 200 calories; no sugar added.

1 protein shake

1 fruit smoothie

1 cup of soup (no potatoes, no heavy cream). Good choices are chicken noodle, vegetable, lentil, chickpea, split pea, black bean, tomato basil, minestrone. Always be careful of sodium content!

BEVERAGES

- Choose one of the following:

Unlimited plain water (flat or fizzy)

1 cup of flavored water

1 cup of lemonade

1 cup of unsweetened iced tea

1 cup of juice (not from concentrate)

12-ounce can of diet soda (no more than 1 per day)

1 cup of low-fat, reduced-fat, or fat-free milk or unsweetened soy or almond milk

MEAL 3

- 1 large green garden salad (3 cups of greens) with 2½ ounces of sliced chicken. You may include a few olives, shredded carrots, and ½ sliced tomato or 5 grape tomatoes. Only 3 tablespoons of fat-free dressing, no bacon bits, no croutons.

BEVERAGES

- Choose one of the following. Try to choose a different beverage from the one you chose in meal 2.

Unlimited plain water (flat or fizzy)

1 cup of flavored water

1 cup of lemonade

1 cup of unsweetened iced tea

1 cup of juice (not from concentrate)

12-ounce can of diet soda (no more than 1 per day)

1 cup of low-fat, reduced-fat, or fat-free milk or unsweetened soy
or almond milk

SNACK 2

- 1 SHRED POP popcorn *or* 1 small scoop of low-fat frozen
  yogurt *or* 3 tablespoons of all-natural granola *or* any other
  item 100 calories or less

Exercise

- **Amount of exercise today:** minimum 40 minutes. If you want to
  do more, all the better! Work as hard as you can! The key is to
  avoid doing steady-state exercise such as walking on the treadmill at the same speed and same incline for a period of time.
  Instead, try to vary your speed, your incline, the distances you
  cover. The goal here is to do high-intensity interval training.
- **Option 1:** Do the *SHRED 27 Burn* workout DVD.
- **Option 2:** Choose two of the cardiovascular exercises below,
  for a total of 40 minutes of exercise.

Walking/running outside or on treadmill

Jogging outside

Elliptical machine

Stationary or mobile bicycle

Swimming laps

Stair climber

200 jump rope revolutions

20-minute treadmill intervals

Zumba or other cardio dance workout

SUPER SHRED WEEK 2, DAY 2

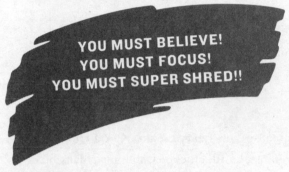

YOU MUST BELIEVE!
YOU MUST FOCUS!
YOU MUST SUPER SHRED!!

MEAL I

- 1 piece of fruit or ½ cup of berries
- Choose one from the following:

1 six-ounce container of low-fat or fat-free yogurt; add fresh fruit

1 egg-white omelet (made with 2 egg whites or ½ cup of Egg Beaters; little butter or cooking spray is allowed)

1 cup of sugar-free cereal with low-fat, reduced-fat, or fat-free milk or unsweetened soy or almond milk

Optional: 1 piece of 100 percent whole-grain or whole-wheat toast

BEVERAGES

- 1 cup of fresh juice (not from concentrate) or 1 cup of low-fat, reduced-fat, or fat-free milk or unsweetened soy or almond milk
- **Optional:** 1 cup of coffee (no more than 1 packet of sugar, 1 tablespoon of milk or half-and-half)

SNACK I

- 1 SHRED BAR *or* any other item 150 calories or less.

MEAL 2

- Choose one of the following. Your choice must not exceed 200 calories; no sugar added.

1 protein shake

1 fruit smoothie

1 cup of soup (no potatoes, no heavy cream). Good choices are chicken noodle, vegetable, lentil, chickpea, split pea, black bean, tomato basil, minestronc. Always be careful of sodium content!

BEVERAGES

- Choose one of the following:

Unlimited plain water (flat or fizzy)

1 cup of flavored water

1 cup of lemonade

1 cup of unsweetened iced tea

1 cup of juice (not from concentrate)

12-ounce can of diet soda (no more than 1 per day)

1 cup of low-fat, reduced-fat, or fat-free milk or unsweetened soy or almond milk

MEAL 3

- 1 cup of brown rice
- 1 cup of cooked beans, chickpeas, or lentils (no baked beans)
- 1 serving of vegetables

BEVERAGES

- Choose one of the following. Try to choose a different beverage from the one you chose in meal 2.

Unlimited plain water (flat or fizzy)

1 cup of flavored water

1 cup of lemonade

1 cup of unsweetened iced tea

1 cup of juice (not from concentrate)

12-ounce can of diet soda (no more than 1 per day)

1 cup of low-fat, reduced-fat, or fat-free milk or unsweetened soy or almond milk

SNACK 2

- 1 SHRED POP popcorn *or* 1 medium cucumber sprinkled with balsamic vinaigrette *or* 9 or 10 black olives *or* any other item 100 calories or less

Exercise

- **Amount of exercise today:** minimum 45 minutes. If you want to do more, all the better! Work as hard as you can! The key is to avoid doing steady-state exercise such as walking on the treadmill at the same speed and same incline for a period of time. Instead, try to vary your speed, your incline, the distances you cover. The goal here is to do high-intensity interval training. Remember, you can always break up the workout. For example, if you don't have time to do it all at once, you can do 25 minutes now and 20 later, or whichever combination works for you.

- **Option 1:** Do the *SHRED 27 Burn* workout DVD and 15 minutes of light weight resistance, using either free weights like dumbbells or resistance bands.
- **Option 2:** Choose two of the cardiovascular exercises below, for a total of 45 minutes of exercise.

Walking/running outside or on treadmill

Jogging outside

Elliptical machine

Stationary or mobile bicycle

Swimming laps

Stair climber

200 jump rope revolutions

20-minute treadmill intervals

Zumba or other cardio dance workout

SUPER SHRED WEEK 2, DAY 3

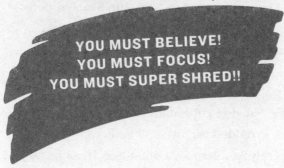

YOU MUST BELIEVE!
YOU MUST FOCUS!
YOU MUST SUPER SHRED!!

MEAL I

- 1 piece of fruit or ½ cup of berries
- Choose from one of the following:

1 pancake the size of a CD with 1 slice of bacon (turkey or pork)

1 grilled cheese sandwich made with 2 slices of regular cheese on 2 slices of 100 percent whole-wheat or whole-grain bread (little butter or cooking spray allowed)

1 cup of sugar-free cereal with low-fat, reduced-fat, or fat-free milk or unsweetened soy or almond milk

1 six-ounce container of low-fat or fat-free yogurt; add fresh fruit

BEVERAGES

- **Must:** 1 cup of water, hot or cold, with 1 tablespoon of freshly squeezed lemon juice
- **Optional:** unlimited plain water
- **Optional:** 1 cup of coffee (no more than 1 packet of sugar, 1 tablespoon of milk or half-and-half)

SNACK I

- 1 SHRED BAR *or* 1 cup of sugar snap peas with 3 tablespoons of hummus *or* 2 squares of graham crackers and 8 ounces of low-fat or skim milk *or* any other item 150 calories or less

MEAL 2

- 1 large green garden salad (4 cups of greens). You may include a few olives, shredded carrots, and ½ sliced tomato or 5 grape tomatoes. Only 3 tablespoons of fat-free dressing, no bacon bits, no croutons.

BEVERAGES

- Choose one of the following:

Unlimited plain water (flat or fizzy)

1 cup of flavored water

1 cup of lemonade

1 cup of unsweetened iced tea

1 cup of juice (not from concentrate)

12-ounce can of diet soda (no more than 1 per day)

1 cup of low-fat, reduced-fat, or fat-free milk or unsweetened soy or almond milk

MEAL 3

- Choose one of the following:

2 chicken fingers

3 servings of veggies with 1 cup of brown rice

6 jumbo shrimp (2 tablespoons cocktail sauce)

1 cup of chicken stir-fry

5-ounce piece of fish (baked or grilled, not fried)

1 serving of veggies if you chose chicken, shrimp, or fish

BEVERAGES

- Choose one of the following. Try to choose a different beverage from the one you chose in meal 2.

Unlimited plain water (flat or fizzy)

1 cup of flavored water

1 cup of lemonade

1 cup of unsweetened iced tea

1 cup of juice (not from concentrate)

12-ounce can of diet soda (no more than 1 per day)

1 cup of low-fat, reduced-fat, or fat-free milk or unsweetened soy or almond milk

SNACK 2

- 1 SHRED POP popcorn *or* 3 ounces of cod, cooked *or* 1 cup of fresh raspberries with dash of cinnamon and 1 teaspoon of honey *or* any other item 100 calories or less

Exercise

- Rest Day! This is a rest day, especially if you are aching and your muscles need recovery. But if you feel up to it and you decide to do some exercise on your own, that is completely allowed. Thirty minutes of cardio training will always serve you well, so feel free to get in some extra work. Each exercise session will move you closer to your goal!

SUPER SHRED WEEK 2, DAY 4

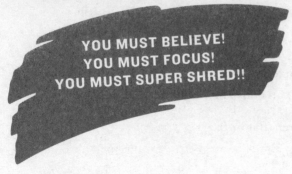

YOU MUST BELIEVE!
YOU MUST FOCUS!
YOU MUST SUPER SHRED!!

MEAL I

- 1 piece of fruit or ½ cup of berries
- Choose one of the following. Make sure it's 200 calories or less; no sugar added.

  1 fruit smoothie

  1 protein shake

BEVERAGES

- **Must:** 1 cup of green tea or 1 cup of hibiscus tea (a dash of sugar is allowed)
- **Optional:** unlimited plain water
- **Optional:** 1 cup of coffee (no more than 1 packet of sugar, 1 tablespoon of milk or half-and-half)

SNACK I

- 1 SHRED BAR *or* 1 cup of grape tomatoes *or* ½ cup of roasted chickpeas *or* any other item 150 calories or less

MEAL 2

- 1 serving of vegetables or 1 small green garden salad (2 cups of greens). You may include a couple of olives, shredded carrots, a couple of small slices of tomato. Only 1 tablespoon of fat-free dressing, no bacon bits, no croutons.

- Choose one of the following:

1 turkey sandwich or 1 chicken sandwich (1 ounce of sliced meat) on 100 percent whole-grain or whole-wheat bread with a teaspoon of mustard or mayo, a slice of tomato, lettuce, and 1 slice of cheese

5 ounces fish (baked or grilled, not fried)

BEVERAGES

- Choose one of the following:

Unlimited plain water (flat or fizzy)

1 cup of flavored water

1 cup of lemonade

1 cup of unsweetened iced tea

1 cup of juice (not from concentrate)

12-ounce can of diet soda (no more than 1 per day)

1 cup of low-fat, reduced-fat, or fat-free milk or unsweetened soy or almond milk

MEAL 3

- 1 cup of soup (no potatoes, no heavy cream). Good choices are chicken noodle, vegetable, lentil, chickpea, split pea, black bean, tomato basil, minestrone. Always be careful of sodium content!

- ½ cup of brown rice
- 1 serving of vegetables

BEVERAGES

- Choose one of the following. Try to choose a different beverage from the one you chose in meal 2.

Unlimited plain water (flat or fizzy)

1 cup of flavored water

1 cup of lemonade

1 cup of unsweetened iced tea

1 cup of juice (not from concentrate)

12-ounce can of diet soda (no more than 1 per day)

1 cup of low-fat, reduced-fat, or fat-free milk or unsweetened soy or almond milk

SNACK 2

- 1 SHRED POP popcorn *or* 1 hard-boiled egg with ½ cup of sugar snap peas *or* ½ cup of fat-free yogurt and ½ cup of blueberries *or* any other item 100 calories or less

Exercise

- **Amount of exercise today:** minimum 40 minutes. If you want to do more, all the better! Work as hard as you can! The key is to avoid doing steady-state exercise such as walking on the treadmill at the same speed and same incline for a period of time. Instead, try to vary your speed, your incline, the distances you cover. The goal here is to do high-intensity interval training.

- **Option 1:** Do the *SHRED 27 Burn* workout DVD.
- **Option 2:** Choose two of the cardiovascular exercises below, for a total of 40 minutes of exercise.

Walking/running outside or on treadmill

Jogging outside

Elliptical machine

Stationary or mobile bicycle

Swimming laps

Stair climber

200 jump rope revolutions

20-minute treadmill intervals

Zumba or other cardio dance workout

SUPER SHRED WEEK 2, DAY 5
SUPER SHREDDER DAY

YOU MUST BELIEVE!
YOU MUST FOCUS!
YOU MUST SUPER SHRED!!

MEAL I
- Choose one of the following. Make sure it's 200 calories or less; no sugar added.

1 fruit smoothie

1 protein shake

BEVERAGES

- **Optional:** unlimited plain water
- **Optional:** 1 cup of coffee or 1 cup of tea (1 packet of sugar, 1 tablespoon of milk or half-and-half)

SNACK I

- 1 SHRED BAR *or* 2 scoops of sorbet *or* 9 chocolate-covered almonds *or* any other item 150 calories or less

MEAL 2

- **Must:** 1 cup of plain water before your meal
- 1½ cups of soup (no potatoes, no heavy cream). Good choices are chicken noodle, vegetable, lentil, chickpea, split pea, black bean, tomato basil, minestrone. Always be careful of sodium content!

BEVERAGES

- Choose one of the following:

Unlimited plain water (flat or fizzy)

1 cup of flavored water

1 cup of lemonade

1 cup of unsweetened iced tea

1 cup of juice (not from concentrate)

12-ounce can of diet soda (no more than 1 per day)

1 cup of low-fat, reduced-fat, or fat-free milk or unsweetened soy or almond milk

MEAL 3

- **Must:** 1 cup of plain water before your meal
- 1½ cups of soup. Try to choose a soup different from the one you had in meal 2. Try to avoid soups made with heavy cream. Good choices are chicken noodle, vegetable, lentil, chickpea, split pea, black bean, tomato basil, minestrone. Always be careful of sodium content!

BEVERAGES

- Choose one of the following. Try to choose a different beverage from the one you chose in meal 2.

Unlimited plain water (flat or fizzy)

1 cup of flavored water

1 cup of lemonade

1 cup of unsweetened iced tea

1 cup of juice (not from concentrate)

12-ounce can of diet soda (no more than 1 per day)

1 cup of low-fat, reduced-fat, or fat-free milk or unsweetened soy or almond milk

SNACK 2

- 1 SHRED POP popcorn *or* 11 blue-corn tortilla chips *or* ½ whole-wheat English muffin topped with 1 teaspoon of fruit butter *or* any other item 100 calories or less

Exercise

- **Amount of exercise today:** minimum 40 minutes. If you want to do more, all the better! Work as hard as you can! The key is to avoid doing steady-state exercise such as walking on the treadmill at the same speed and same incline for a period of time. Instead, try to vary your speed, your incline, the distances you cover. The goal here is to do high-intensity interval training. If necessary, you can always break up your workout into two different sessions.
- **Option 1:** Do the *SHRED 27 Burn* workout DVD.
- **Option 2:** Choose two of the cardiovascular exercises below, for a total of 40 minutes of exercise.

Walking/running outside or on treadmill

Jogging outside

Elliptical machine

Stationary or mobile bicycle

Swimming laps

Stair climber

200 jump rope revolutions

20-minute treadmill intervals

Zumba or other cardio dance workout

SUPER SHRED WEEK 2, DAY 6

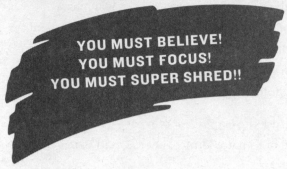

YOU MUST BELIEVE!
YOU MUST FOCUS!
YOU MUST SUPER SHRED!!

MEAL I

- 1 piece of fruit or ½ cup of berries.
- Choose one of the following:

1 cup of sugar-free cereal with low-fat, reduced-fat, or fat-free milk or unsweetened soy or almond milk

1 cup of oatmeal

1 cup of grits

1 six-ounce container of low-fat or fat-free yogurt; add fresh fruit

BEVERAGES

- **Optional:** unlimited plain water
- **Optional:** 1 cup of coffee (no more than 1 packet of sugar, 1 tablespoon of milk or half-and-half) or 1 cup of tea or 1 cup of fresh juice (not from concentrate)

SNACK I

- 1 SHRED BAR *or* 1 cup of grapes with 10 almonds *or* ½ cup of frozen banana slices *or* any other item 150 calories or less.

MEAL 2

- 1 small green garden salad (2 cups of greens). You may include a couple of olives, shredded carrots, a couple of small slices of tomato. Only 1 tablespoon of fat-free dressing, no bacon bits, no croutons.
- Choose one of the following:

4-ounce hamburger (use the leanest cut of meat—ground sirloin) on a bun with a slice of tomato, lettuce, cheese, and ½ teaspoon of ketchup optional

4-ounce veggie burger on a bun with a slice of tomato, lettuce, cheese, and ½ teaspoon of ketchup optional

4-ounce turkey burger on a bun with a slice of tomato, lettuce, cheese, and ½ teaspoon of ketchup optional

1 cup of soup (no potatoes, no heavy cream). Good choices are chicken noodle, vegetable, lentil, chickpea, split pea, black bean, tomato basil, minestrone. Always be careful of sodium content!

BEVERAGES

- Choose one of the following:

Unlimited plain water (flat or fizzy)

1 cup of flavored water

1 cup of lemonade

1 cup of unsweetened iced tea

1 cup of juice (not from concentrate)

12-ounce can of diet soda (no more than 1 per day)

1 cup of low-fat, reduced-fat, or fat-free milk or unsweetened soy or almond milk

MEAL 3

- 2 servings of vegetables
- Choose one of the following:

5-ounce piece of chicken (no skin, baked or grilled, not fried)

5-ounce piece of turkey (no skin, not fried)

5-ounce piece of ham

5-ounce turkey burger

BEVERAGES

- Choose one of the following. Try to choose a different beverage from the one you chose in meal 2.

Unlimited plain water (flat or fizzy)

1 cup of flavored water

1 cup of lemonade

1 cup of unsweetened iced tea

1 cup of juice (not from concentrate)

12-ounce can of diet soda (no more than 1 per day)

1 cup of low-fat, reduced-fat, or fat-free milk or unsweetened soy or almond milk

SNACK 2

- 1 SHRED POP popcorn *or* 1 raw large carrot *or* 25 oil-roasted peanuts *or* any other item 100 calories or less

Exercise

- **Amount of exercise today:** minimum 40 minutes. If you want to do more, all the better! Work as hard as you can! The key is to avoid doing steady-state exercise such as walking on the treadmill at the same speed and same incline for a period of time. Instead, try to vary your speed, your incline, the distances you cover. The goal here is to do high-intensity interval training.
- **Option 1:** Do the *SHRED 27 Burn* workout DVD.
- **Option 2:** Choose two of the cardiovascular exercises below, for a total of 40 minutes of exercise.

Walking/running outside or on treadmill

Jogging outside

Elliptical machine

Stationary or mobile bicycle

Swimming laps

Stair climber

200 jump rope revolutions

20-minute treadmill intervals

Zumba or other cardio dance workout

SUPER SHRED WEEK 2, DAY 7

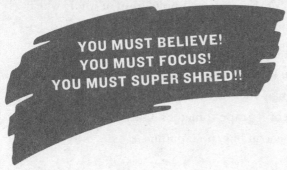

YOU MUST BELIEVE!
YOU MUST FOCUS!
YOU MUST SUPER SHRED!!

MEAL 1

- 1 piece of fruit or ½ cup of berries
- Choose one of the following. Your choice must be
  200 calories or less; no sugar added.

1 fruit smoothie

1 protein shake

BEVERAGES

- **Optional:** unlimited plain water
- **Optional:** 1 cup of coffee (no more than 1 packet of sugar, 1
  tablespoon of milk or half-and-half) or 1 cup of tea or 1 cup
  of fresh juice (not from concentrate)

SNACK 1

- 1 SHRED BAR *or* 1 can of tuna, drained and seasoned to
  taste, *or* 25 frozen red seedless grapes *or* any other item
  150 calories or less

MEAL 2

- Choose one of the following:

1 turkey sandwich or 1 chicken sandwich (1 ounce of sliced turkey or chicken meat) on 100 percent whole-grain or whole-wheat bread with a teaspoon of mustard or mayo, a slice of tomato, lettuce, and 1 slice of cheese

1 large green garden salad (3 cups of greens) with 2½ ounces of sliced chicken. You may include a few olives, shredded carrots, and ½ sliced tomato or 5 grape tomatoes. Only 3 tablespoons of fat-free dressing, no bacon bits, no croutons.

BEVERAGES

- Choose one of the following:

Unlimited plain water (flat or fizzy)

1 cup of flavored water

1 cup of lemonade

1 cup of unsweetened iced tea

1 cup of juice (not from concentrate)

12-ounce can of diet soda (no more than 1 per day)

1 cup of low-fat, reduced-fat, or fat-free milk or unsweetened soy or almond milk

MEAL 3

- 1 serving of vegetables
- Choose one of the following:

1 cup of pasta with marinara sauce (no cream sauce)

5-ounce piece of fish (baked or grilled, not fried)

5-ounce piece of chicken (no skin, baked or grilled, not fried)

BEVERAGES

- Choose one of the following. Try to choose a different beverage from the one you chose in meal 2.

Unlimited plain water (flat or fizzy)

1 cup of flavored water

1 cup of lemonade

1 cup of unsweetened iced tea

1 cup of juice (not from concentrate)

12-ounce can of diet soda (no more than 1 per day)

1 cup of low-fat, reduced-fat, or fat-free milk or unsweetened soy or almond milk

SNACK 2

- 1 SHRED POP popcorn *or* 1 cup of low-fat salsa with 10 tortilla chips *or* 1 low-fat mozzarella cheese stick with small sliced apple *or* any other item 100 calories or less

Exercise

- Rest Day! This is a rest day, especially if you are aching and your muscles need recovery. But if you feel up to it and you decide to do some exercise on your own, that is completely allowed. Thirty minutes of cardio training will always serve you well, so feel free to get in some extra work. Each exercise session will move you closer to your goal!

CHAPTER 5

Week 3: Shape

Congrats on making it to the third leg of our four-week journey! Making it this far is a testament to your drive and determination. You have asked a lot of your body and mind and they are delivering. Now that we're halfway through the program, it's time to shape our bodies. This week you will push yourself harder than ever. You must have complete dedication, focus, and a sense of humor this week. This is meant to be a tough week, but it's only seven days. You can do almost *anything* for seven days. Remind yourself every morning when you get up and every night when you go to sleep that this is something you *can* and *must* and *will* do. Mental toughness has never been more important than it is this week.

So far, you have lost a considerable amount of weight in a short period of time. That means you have mobilized a lot of those plump fat cells and burned the energy they had been storing, causing them to shrink. Now we want to start shaping the body. Your arms, legs, and midsection can begin to take on the form that you desire.

Are you going to have a six-pack overnight? No. But you will likely be down at least one clothing size and in some cases maybe even two sizes, as your pants and tops should now be fitting more loosely. Your body is responding to your hard work and the payoff at the end of this week will be quite visible. You might see it in your jawline, your neck, or your inner thighs. You and others *will* notice a difference. Remember: all of this starts—and continues—with hard work.

Your meal plan this week will be drastically different from those of the last two weeks. You will now have only two meals a day, but your snacks will increase to four. Snacks remain optional but are strongly recommended. You are allowed to have a "floating bonus snack." This is an extra snack in addition to what is written in the daily menu. It can be eaten at any time of the day, but it must be 100 calories or less. Use this snack only if you need it. It's meant to be an emergency relief if your body really needs it.

This is the week of calorie disruption we discussed in chapter 1. The goal here is to challenge your body so that it's off kilter, constantly guessing what food it will be seeing next and what exercise challenges it will face. Here is a sample eating schedule:

7:30 A.M.	8:30 A.M.	10:30 A.M.	12:30 P.M.	2:30 P.M.	5:30 P.M.	7:00 P.M.
Awake	Meal 1	Snack 1	Snack 2	Snack 3	Meal 2	Snack 4

SUPER SHRED Week 3 Grocery List

This is a list that takes into consideration the different combinations of food and beverage items offered to you this week. Because the program has a lot of flexibility and choices, no one list can be constructed for everyone. Note that there are some items that you *must* have. Be sure to buy them to have on hand when the program calls for them. If you are a vegetarian, you don't need to eat the meat meals. Make appropriate substitutions, but be mindful of calorie counts.

FRUIT

- **Must:** 6 servings of fruit. This can be a combination of fruits such as berries, apples, bananas, pineapple, etc.
- **Optional:** 2 servings of fresh fruit for low-fat yogurt
- **Serving size:** 1 piece of fruit = 1 serving; ½ cup of berries = 1 serving

BREAKFAST OPTIONS

- 5 breakfast meals: Choose your combination from this list.

4 cups oatmeal (1 cup cooked = 1 meal)

3 cups of Cream of Wheat or farina (1 cup cooked = 1 meal)

5 cups sugar-free or low-sugar (under 5 grams) dry cereal (1 cup = 1 meal)

9 eggs

1 cup Egg Beaters

1 loaf of bread

2 pancakes the size of a CD

2 strips of bacon (turkey or bacon)

3 six-ounce containers of low-fat plain yogurt

1 grilled cheese sandwich made with 2 slices of regular cheese on 2 pieces of 100 percent whole-grain or whole-wheat bread

1 cup of grits (1 cup cooked = 1 meal; instant is allowed)

BEVERAGES

- **Must:** 19 drink options for the week. Water is not included; you may have as much as you want. Choose your combinations from the list below. Then purchase your choices for the week.

11 cups of fresh juice

14 cups of coffee

7 twelve-ounce cans of diet soda

12 cups of low-fat, reduced-fat, or fat-free milk or unsweetened soy or almond milk

7 cups of unsweetened iced tea

6 cups of lemonade

7 cups of flavored water

SALADS

- **Must:** 1 large green garden salad
- **Optional:** You will have other opportunities to have salads. Those opportunities are listed below. You should choose which of these you want, then purchase accordingly.

3 large green garden salads

VEGETABLES

- **Must:** 10 servings
- **Optional:** 2 servings. You will have other vegetable opportunities. If you choose them, purchase accordingly.
- **Serving size:** 1 serving is approximately the size of your fist

MEAT AND FISH

- **Must:** 6 servings. Choose from the list below. But note the maximum number of servings you may have for each option.
- **Optional:** 4 servings
- **Serving size:** 1 serving = 5 ounces, approximately the size of a deck and a half of playing cards, once cooked.
- Your maximum number of servings for the week will be 6 if you choose all of the optional servings. Make your choices from the list below, mixing them up. Remember, you must have at least 2 servings.

6 six-ounce pieces of chicken (skinless)

5 five-ounce pieces of turkey

5 five-ounce pieces of fish

3 two-and-a-half-ounce slices of roasted chicken

SNACKS

- Choose 28 snacks for the entire week, such as nuts, Popsicles, chocolate-covered strawberries, and other items listed in chapter 7.

14 SHRED BARs or other snack items 150 calories or less

14 Bags SHRED POP popcorn or other snack items 100 calories or less

SMOOTHIES, PROTEIN SHAKES

- **Must:** 2 servings from the items listed below. Each item must be 200 calories or less, with no added sugar. Choose the combination that you desire and purchase ingredients accordingly.

2 fruit smoothies

2 protein shakes

OPTIONAL MEAL CHOICES

- Throughout the week you will have the opportunity to have the meals listed below. Choose which of them you want, then purchase accordingly. You can choose all or none of them.

2 cups of pasta

2 slices of small cheese pizza (no larger than 5 inches across the crust and 5 inches long)

1 serving of lasagna, with or without meat (4 inches × 3 inches × 1 inch)

1 veggie burger (3 inches in diameter, ½ inch thick)

EXTRAS

- These are things you might want to have during the week, so stock up on them.

Low-fat grated cheese for omelets

Diced vegetables for omelets

Half-and-half

Extra milk for cereal and coffee

Salad toppings

Fat-free dressing for salad

SUPER SHRED Week 3 Guidelines

- Weigh yourself in the morning the day you start the program and make sure you record it. You will weigh yourself only once a week, so even if you are tempted, stay off the scale. Your body naturally fluctuates a couple of pounds from day to day. Measuring yourself every day could give you an inaccurate weight and unnecessarily stress you and lead you to believe you're not succeeding. Your next weigh-in will be exactly a week from now. Make sure you weigh yourself in the same manner each time: if you weighed in wearing certain clothes or no clothes at all, make sure you do the same this time around and as close to the same time of the day. Make sure you use the same scale each time, as different scales can be off by several pounds, thus destroying the accuracy of your measure.

• Do not skip meals. Even if you're not hungry, just have something during the allotted time. You can always grab a piece of fruit or something small during your mealtime. Also, you don't have to eat all of the meal. You can eat just some of it. If you're not hungry, don't stuff yourself. Just eat a little. The key is to eat at regularly scheduled times so that your body grows accustomed to these eating times. Each week will change, so it's important to quickly adapt to the week that you're in and its related schedule. During the course of the week you should never go more than 4 hours without eating something. Your meals should be 3 to 4 hours apart. Your snacks should fall about 1½ hours after meals. If you miss a meal or snack, you can't save it and eat it later or combine them. Once that time has passed, move on and hit your next mark.

• All of your shakes and smoothies this week must be 200 calories or less, with no added sugar. If you follow the recipes in the back of the book, they will fit this description. If you buy them from a store, be sure of the calorie count. Also, be mindful of the serving sizes of the drinks. If the recipe makes more than one serving, be sure you drink only one at a time. If the store-bought product contains more than 1 serving, just drink the equivalent of 1 serving and refrigerate the rest for next time.

- Snacks are optional, but highly recommended, especially for this week. The SHRED BARs and SHRED POP popcorn are suggested for many of your snacks, as they are specifically made with all of the nutritional guidelines in mind. However, you may have other snacks as long as they fall under the proper calorie count.

- Soups are an option, including store-bought soups. But make sure you look at the sodium content: no more than 480 milligrams *per serving*. Be mindful of the serving size. For the purpose of this plan, 1 serving is equivalent to 1 cup, whether you eat store-bought soup or make it fresh. You may have 1 saltine cracker with your soup.

- Consume 1 cup of water before *every* meal and *every* snack. This is critical this week.

- You are allowed 2 cups of coffee each day, 1 cup at breakfast. Stay away from all those fancy coffee preparations—lattes, Frappuccinos, coffees that pile on the calories. A tablespoon of sugar and a little half-and-half or milk won't hurt, but don't go overboard.

- Canned and frozen fruits and vegetables are allowed. Please be aware of added ingredients. Make sure they are either packed in water or labeled "no sugar added." The key is to have food in its most natural state with the least amount of processing. Make sure you check the sodium levels, as they can be quite high: try to keep the amount to 480 milligrams of salt for any serving of food.

- While fresh-squeezed juice is definitely preferred, you can drink store-bought juice. Just make sure it says "not from concentrate" and "no sugar added." If you're a diabetic or have trouble regulating your blood sugar, choose a different beverage option, such as water, milk, or tea.

- No alcohol this week. This is a clean week. Save your calories for something with important nutrients that makes you feel full.

- You are allowed 1 diet soda per day if you desire. Regular soda is not recommended.

- Do not eat your last meal within 90 minutes of going to sleep. If because of circumstances you're eating late and know you're going right to bed, then consume half the meal.

- Spices are unlimited, so enjoy. Salt is not a spice. You are allowed to add no more than ½ teaspoon of salt to your food each day.

- If you are a vegetarian or diabetic or need to avoid certain foods owing to other medical conditions, it is completely acceptable to make substitutions. But make smart substitutions and be mindful of the portion sizes.

- Serving sizes: A 5-ounce serving of fish or meat after being cooked is typically the size of a deck and a half of playing cards. A serving of vegetables is typically the size of an adult's fist. A serving size of hot cereal is 1 cup of *cooked* cereal.

- You may have ½ pat of butter (about ½ teaspoon) with hot cereal.

- You may have 1 teaspoon of sugar (white or brown) or ½ teaspoon of honey with hot or cold cereals.

- If you must switch days or meals within a day for scheduling reasons, try to do so as infrequently as possible.

- If you need to rearrange your exercise regimen for scheduling reasons, it is permissible to do so.

- **Floating Bonus Snack.** This week you are allowed 1 extra snack of 100 calories or less any time throughout the day when you feel like you absolutely need it. Be strategic about this snack. If you really don't need it, don't use it. But if you are feeling like your body is simply shutting down or the hunger pangs are too intense, then by all means treat yourself to this snack.

SUPER SHRED WEEK 3, DAY 1

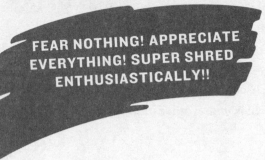

FEAR NOTHING! APPRECIATE EVERYTHING! SUPER SHRED ENTHUSIASTICALLY!!

Note: Don't forget that you're allowed a Floating Bonus Snack today!

MEAL I

- 1 piece of fruit. Choose from the following, though you can choose others: pear, apple, ½ cup of raspberries or strawberries or blueberries or blackberries, ½ grapefruit, ½ cup of cherries.
- Choose one of the following:

  2 pancakes the size of a CD with 2 strips of bacon (pork or turkey)

  2 scrambled eggs (diced veggie and 1 tablespoon shredded cheese optional; little butter or cooking spray allowed)

  1 egg-white omelet (2 egg whites or ½ cup Egg Beaters; diced veggies optional)

  1 cup of oatmeal

  1 cup of sugar-free cereal with low-fat, reduced-fat, or fat-free milk or unsweetened soy or almond milk

BEVERAGES

- **Must:** 1 cup of fresh juice (not from concentrate) *or* 1 cup of low-fat, reduced-fat, or fat-free milk or unsweetened soy or almond milk

- **Optional:** unlimited plain water
- **Optional:** 1 cup of coffee (no more than 1 packet of sugar, 1 tablespoon of milk or half-and-half)

SNACK 1

- 1 SHRED BAR *or* ½ cup roasted pumpkin seeds *or* 10 baked whole-wheat pita chips *or* any other item 150 calories or less

SNACK 2

- 1 SHRED POP popcorn *or* 1½ cups of puffed rice *or* 1 cup of broccoli florets with 2 tablespoons of dip *or* any other item 100 calories or less

SNACK 3

- Any item 150 calories or less

MEAL 2

- 2 servings of vegetables
- Choose one of the following:

5-ounce piece of chicken (baked or grilled, not fried, no skin)

5-ounce piece of turkey (baked or grilled, not fried, no skin)

5-ounce piece of fish (baked or grilled, not fried)

BEVERAGES

- Choose one of the following:

Unlimited plain water (flat or fizzy)

1 cup of flavored water

1 cup of lemonade

1 cup of unsweetened iced tea

1 cup of juice (not from concentrate)

12-ounce can of diet soda (no more than 1 per day)

1 cup of low-fat, reduced-fat, or fat-free milk or unsweetened soy or almond milk

SNACK 4

- 1 SHRED POP popcorn *or* any other item 100 calories or less

Exercise

- **Amount of exercise today:** minimum 40 minutes. If you want to do more, all the better! Work as hard as you can! The key is to avoid doing steady-state exercise such as walking on the treadmill at the same speed and same incline for a period of time. Instead, try to vary your speed, your incline, the distances you cover. The goal here is to do high-intensity interval training. Add 15 minutes of resistance training on this day. You can do free weights or bands. Do this in addition to the cardio.
- **Option 1:** Do the *SHRED 27 Burn* workout DVD.
- **Option 2:** Choose two of the cardiovascular exercises below, for a total of 40 minutes of exercise.

Walking/running outside or on treadmill

Jogging outside

Elliptical machine

Stationary or mobile bicycle

Swimming laps

Stair climber

200 jump rope revolutions

20-minute treadmill intervals

Zumba or other cardio dance workout

SUPER SHRED WEEK 3, DAY 2

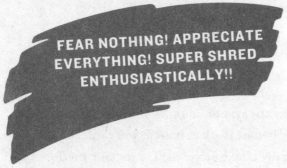

FEAR NOTHING! APPRECIATE EVERYTHING! SUPER SHRED ENTHUSIASTICALLY!!

Note: Don't forget that you're allowed a Floating Bonus Snack today!

MEAL 1

- 1 piece of fruit or ½ cup of berries
- Choose one from the following:

1 cup of oatmeal

1 cup of Cream of Wheat or farina

1 cup of sugar-free cereal with low-fat, reduced-fat, or fat-free milk or unsweetened soy or almond milk

1 six-ounce container of low-fat or fat-free yogurt; add fresh fruit

BEVERAGES

- **Must:** 1 cup of fresh juice (not from concentrate) or 1 cup of low-fat, reduced-fat, or fat-free milk or unsweetened soy or almond milk

- **Optional:** unlimited plain water
- **Optional:** 1 cup of coffee (no more than 1 packet of sugar, 1 tablespoon of milk or half-and-half)

SNACK 1
- 1 SHRED BAR *or* 5 Ritz crackers *or* ½ blueberry muffin *or* any snack item 150 calories or less

SNACK 2
- 1 SHRED POP popcorn *or* 10 baby carrots with 2 tablespoons of low-fat hummus *or* ½ frozen banana dipped in chocolate *or* any snack item 100 calories or less

SNACK 3
- Any snack item 150 calories or less

MEAL 2
- 2 servings of vegetables
- Choose one of the following:

2 slices of small cheese pizza (no larger than 5 inches across the crust and 5 inches long)

1 serving of lasagna (with or without meat), 4 inches × 3 inches × 1 inch

1 veggie burger (3 inches in diameter, ½ inch thick)

6 ounces of turkey or chicken (baked or grilled, not fried, no skin)

BEVERAGES

- Choose one of the following:

Unlimited plain water (flat or fizzy)

1 cup of flavored water

1 cup of lemonade

1 cup of unsweetened iced tea

1 cup of juice (not from concentrate)

12-ounce can of diet soda (no more than 1 per day)

1 cup of low-fat, reduced-fat, or fat-free milk or unsweetened soy or almond milk

SNACK 4

- 1 SHRED POP popcorn *or* 2 ounces of smoked salmon *or* 6 oysters *or* any snack item 100 calories or less

Exercise

- **Amount of exercise today:** minimum 40 minutes. If you want to do more, all the better! Work as hard as you can! The key is to avoid doing steady-state exercise such as walking on the treadmill at the same speed and same incline for a period of time. Instead, try to vary your speed, your incline, the distances you cover. The goal here is to do high-intensity interval training.
- **Option 1:** Do the *SHRED 27 Burn* workout DVD.
- **Option 2:** Choose two of the cardiovascular exercises below, for a total of 40 minutes of exercise.

Walking/running outside or on treadmill

Jogging outside

Elliptical machine

Stationary or mobile bicycle

Swimming laps

Stair climber

200 jump rope revolutions

20-minute treadmill intervals

Zumba or other cardio dance workout

SUPER SHRED WEEK 3, DAY 3
SUPER SHREDDER DAY

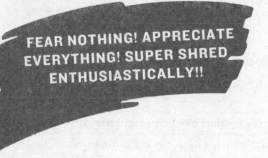

FEAR NOTHING! APPRECIATE EVERYTHING! SUPER SHRED ENTHUSIASTICALLY!!

Note: Don't forget that you're allowed a Floating Bonus Snack today!

MEAL I

- 1 piece of fruit. Choose from the following, though you can choose others: pear, apple, ½ cup of raspberries or strawberries or blueberries or blackberries, ½ grapefruit, ½ cup of cherries.

- Choose one of the following. Your choice must be 200 calories or less; no sugar added.

1 fruit smoothie

1 protein shake

BEVERAGES
- **Optional:** unlimited plain water
- **Optional:** 1 cup of coffee (no more than 1 packet of sugar, 1 tablespoon of milk or half-and-half)

SNACK 1
- Any item 150 calories or less

SNACK 2
- Any item 100 calories or less

SNACK 3
- Any item 150 calories or less

MEAL 2
- 1 large green garden salad (3 cups of greens) with 2½ ounces of sliced chicken. You may include a few olives, shredded carrots, and ½ sliced tomato or 5 grape tomatoes. Only 3 tablespoons of fat-free dressing, no bacon bits, no croutons.

BEVERAGES
- Choose one of the following:

Unlimited plain water (flat or fizzy)

1 cup of flavored water

1 cup of unsweetened iced tea

12-ounce can of diet soda (no more than 1 per day)

1 cup of low-fat, reduced-fat, or fat-free milk or unsweetened soy or almond milk

SNACK 4

- Any other item 100 calories or less

Exercise

- **Amount of exercise today:** minimum 40 minutes. If you want to do more, all the better! Work as hard as you can! The key is to avoid doing steady-state exercise such as walking on the treadmill at the same speed and same incline for a period of time. Instead, try to vary your speed, your incline, the distances you cover. The goal here is to do high-intensity interval training.
- **Option 1:** Do the *SHRED 27 Burn* workout DVD.
- **Option 2:** Choose two of the cardiovascular exercises below, for a total of 40 minutes of exercise.

Walking/running outside or on treadmill

Jogging outside

Elliptical machine

Stationary or mobile bicycle

Swimming laps

Stair climber

200 jump rope revolutions

20-minute treadmill intervals

Zumba or other cardio dance workout

SUPER SHRED WEEK 3, DAY 4

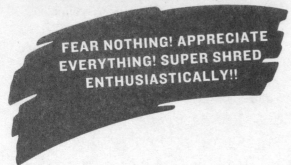

FEAR NOTHING! APPRECIATE EVERYTHING! SUPER SHRED ENTHUSIASTICALLY!!

Note: Don't forget that you're allowed a Floating Bonus Snack today!

MEAL I
- 1 piece of fruit or ½ cup of berries.
- Choose from one of the following:

1 six-ounce container of low-fat or fat-free yogurt; add fresh fruit

2 pieces of whole-grain toast (½ pat butter or ½ teaspoon jelly)

1 scrambled egg (with cooked diced veggies optional, 1 table-spoon of grated cheese allowed; little butter or cooking spray)

1 cup of sugar-free cereal with low-fat, reduced-fat, or fat-free milk or unsweetened soy or almond milk

BEVERAGES
- **Must:** 1 cup of fresh juice (not from concentrate) *or* 1 cup of low-fat or fat-free milk or unsweetened soy or almond milk
- **Optional:** unlimited plain water
- **Optional:** 1 cup of coffee (no more than 1 packet of sugar, 1 tablespoon of milk or half-and-half)

SNACK 1

- 1 SHRED BAR *or* 7 olives stuffed with blue cheese *or* 1 small baked potato topped with 1 tablespoon of salsa *or* any other item 150 calories or less

SNACK 2

- 1 SHRED POP popcorn *or* 20 grapes with 15 peanuts *or* 2 slices of deli turkey breast *or* any snack item 100 calories or less

SNACK 3

- 1 SHRED BAR *or* 1 cup of cherries *or* 2 Fudgsicles *or* any snack item 150 calories or less

MEAL 2

- 2 servings of vegetables
- Choose one of the following:

5-ounce piece of chicken (baked or grilled, not fried, no skin)

5-ounce piece of fish (baked or grilled, not fried)

5-ounce piece of turkey (baked, not fried, no skin)

BEVERAGES

- Choose one of the following:

Unlimited plain water (flat or fizzy)

1 cup of flavored water

1 cup of lemonade

1 cup of unsweetened iced tea

1 cup of juice (not from concentrate)

12-ounce can of diet soda (no more than 1 per day)

1 cup of low-fat, reduced-fat, or fat-free milk or unsweetened soy
or almond milk

SNACK 4
- 1 SHRED POP popcorn or any snack item 100 calories or less

Exercise

- Rest Day! This is a rest day, especially if you are aching and
  your muscles need recovery. But if you feel up to it and you
  decide to do some exercise on your own, that is completely
  allowed. Thirty minutes of cardio training will always serve
  you well, so feel free to get in some extra work. Each exercise
  session will move you closer to your goal!

SUPER SHRED WEEK 3, DAY 5

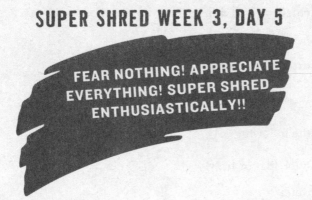

FEAR NOTHING! APPRECIATE
EVERYTHING! SUPER SHRED
ENTHUSIASTICALLY!!

Note: Don't forget that you're allowed a Floating Bonus Snack
today!

MEAL I

- 1 piece of fruit. Choose from the following, though you can choose others: pear, apple, ½ cup of raspberries or strawberries or blueberries or blackberries, ½ grapefruit, ½ cup of cherries.
- Choose one of the following. Your choice must be 200 calories or less; no sugar added.

1 fruit smoothie

1 protein shake

BEVERAGES

- **Optional:** unlimited plain water
- **Optional:** 1 cup of coffee (no more than 1 packet of sugar, 1 tablespoon of milk or half-and-half)

SNACK I

- 1 SHRED BAR *or* 1 cup of grape tomatoes *or* 1½ cups of fruit salad *or* any snack item 150 calories or less

SNACK 2

- 1 SHRED POP popcorn *or* 8 small shrimp with 3 tablespoons of cocktail sauce *or* ½ cup of low-fat salsa with 10 tortilla chips *or* any snack item 100 calories or less

SNACK 3

- 1 SHRED BAR *or* 4 chocolate chip cookies the size of a poker chip *or* ½ cup of roasted chickpeas *or* any snack item 150 calories or less

MEAL 2

- 2 servings of vegetables
- Choose one of the following. Make sure it is different from yesterday's second meal.

5-ounce piece of chicken (baked or grilled, not fried, no skin)

5-ounce piece of turkey (not fried, no skin)

5-ounce piece of fish (baked or grilled, not fried)

1 large green garden salad (3 cups of greens) with 2½ ounces of sliced chicken. You may include a few olives, shredded carrots, and ½ sliced tomato or 5 grape tomatoes. Only 3 tablespoons of fat-free dressing, no bacon bits, no croutons.

1 cup of whole-grain pasta with marinara sauce (ground meat optional)

BEVERAGES

- Choose one of the following:

Unlimited plain water (flat or fizzy)

1 cup of flavored water

1 cup of lemonade

1 cup of unsweetened iced tea

1 cup of juice (not from concentrate)

12-ounce can of diet soda (no more than 1 per day)

1 cup of low-fat, reduced-fat, *or* fat-free milk or unsweetened soy or almond milk

SNACK 4

- 1 SHRED POP popcorn *or* any other item 100 calories or less

Exercise

- **Amount of exercise today:** minimum 50 minutes. If you want to do more, all the better! Work as hard as you can! The key is to avoid doing steady-state exercise such as walking on the treadmill at the same speed and same incline for a period of time. Instead, try to vary your speed, your incline, the distances you cover. The goal here is to do high-intensity interval training. Add 15 minutes of resistance training on this day. You can do free weights or bands. Do this in addition to the cardio.
- **Option 1:** Do the full *SHRED 27 Burn* workout DVD twice. Do this in two separate sessions at least 4 hours apart.
- **Option 2:** Choose two of the cardiovascular exercises below, for a total of 50 minutes of exercise. You can do this in two separate sessions.

Walking/running outside or on treadmill

Jogging outside

Elliptical machine

Stationary or mobile bicycle

Swimming laps

Stair climber

200 jump rope revolutions

20-minute treadmill intervals

Zumba or other cardio dance workout

SUPER SHRED WEEK 3, DAY 6

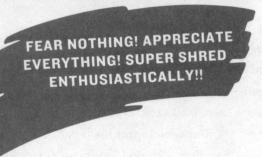

FEAR NOTHING! APPRECIATE EVERYTHING! SUPER SHRED ENTHUSIASTICALLY!!

Note: Don't forget that you're allowed a Floating Bonus Snack today!

MEAL I

- 1 piece of fruit. Choose from the following, though you can choose others: pear, apple, ½ cup of raspberries or strawberries or blueberries or blackberries, ½ grapefruit, ½ cup of cherries.

- Choose one of the following:

  2 scrambled eggs (diced veggie and 1 tablespoon shredded cheese optional; little butter or cooking spray allowed)

  1 egg-white omelet (2 egg whites or ½ cup Egg Beaters; diced veggies optional)

  1 cup of oatmeal

  1 cup of sugar-free cereal with low-fat, reduced-fat, or fat-free milk or unsweetened soy or almond milk

  1 grilled cheese sandwich made with 2 slices of regular cheese on 2 slices of 100 percent whole-wheat or whole-grain bread (little butter or cooking spray allowed)

BEVERAGES

- **Must:** 1 cup of fresh juice (not from concentrate) or 1 cup of low-fat, reduced-fat, or fat-free milk or unsweetened soy or almond milk
- **Optional:** unlimited plain water
- **Optional:** 1 cup of coffee (no more than 1 packet of sugar, 1 tablespoon of milk or half-and-half)

SNACK 1

- Any snack item 150 calories or less

SNACK 2

- Any snack item 100 calories or less

SNACK 3

- Any snack item 150 calories or less

MEAL 2

- 2 servings of vegetables
- Choose one of the following. Make sure it is different from the previous day's second meal.

5-ounce piece of chicken (baked or grilled, not fried, no skin)

5-ounce piece of turkey (not fried, no skin)

5-ounce piece of fish (baked or grilled, not fried)

1 large green garden salad (3 cups of greens) with 2½ ounces of sliced chicken. You may include a few olives, shredded carrots, and ½ sliced tomato or 5 grape tomatoes. Only 3 tablespoons of fat-free dressing, no bacon bits, no croutons.

1 cup of whole-grain pasta with marinara sauce (ground meat optional)

BEVERAGES

- Choose one of the following:

Unlimited plain water (flat or fizzy)

1 cup of flavored water

1 cup of lemonade

1 cup of unsweetened iced tea

1 cup of juice (not from concentrate)

12-ounce can of diet soda (no more than 1 per day)

1 cup of low-fat, reduced-fat, or fat-free milk or unsweetened soy or almond milk

SNACK 4

- Any snack item 100 calories or less

Exercise

- **Amount of exercise today:** minimum 40 minutes. If you want to do more, all the better! Work as hard as you can! The key is to avoid doing steady-state exercise such as walking on the treadmill at the same speed and same incline for a period of time. Instead, try to vary your speed, your incline, the distances you cover. The goal here is to do high-intensity interval training. Add 15 minutes of resistance training on this day. You can do free weights or bands. Do this in addition to the cardio.
- **Option 1:** Do the *SHRED 27 Burn* workout DVD.
- **Option 2:** Choose two of the cardiovascular exercises below, for a total of 40 minutes of exercise.

Walking/running outside or on treadmill

Jogging outside

Elliptical machine

Stationary or mobile bicycle

Swimming laps

Stair climber

200 jump rope revolutions

20-minute treadmill intervals

Zumba or other cardio dance workout

SUPER SHRED WEEK 3, DAY 7

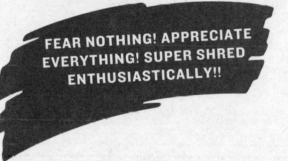

FEAR NOTHING! APPRECIATE EVERYTHING! SUPER SHRED ENTHUSIASTICALLY!!

Note: Don't forget that you're allowed a Floating Bonus Snack today!

MEAL I

- 1 piece of fruit. Choose from the following, though you can choose others: pear, apple, ½ cup of raspberries or strawberries or blueberries or blackberries, ½ grapefruit, ½ cup of cherries.
- Choose one of the following:

1 cup of oatmeal

1 cup of sugar-free cereal with low-fat, reduced-fat, or fat-free milk or unsweetened soy or almond milk

1 cup of grits

1 cup of Cream of Wheat or farina

1 six-ounce container of low-fat or fat-free yogurt; add fresh fruit

BEVERAGES

- **Must:** 1 cup of fresh juice (not from concentrate) or 1 cup of low-fat, reduced-fat, or fat-free milk or unsweetened almond or soy milk
- **Optional:** unlimited plain water
- **Optional:** 1 cup of coffee (no more than 1 packet of sugar, 1 tablespoon of milk or half-and-half)

SNACK 1

- 1 SHRED BAR *or* 1 cup of grape tomatoes *or* 1 medium sliced red bell pepper with ¼ cup of guacamole *or* any other item 150 calories or less

SNACK 2

- 1 SHRED POP popcorn *or* 6 dried apricots *or* 3 crackers lightly spread with peanut butter *or* any other item 100 calories or less

SNACK 3

- 1 SHRED BAR *or* 1 medium mango *or* ½ cup of shelled pistachios *or* any other item 150 calories or less

MEAL 2

- 2 servings of vegetables (only if you don't choose the salad option below)
- Choose one of the following:

5-ounce piece of chicken (baked or grilled, not fried, no skin)

5-ounce piece of turkey (not fried, no skin)

5-ounce piece of fish (baked or grilled, not fried)

1 large green garden salad (3 cups of greens) with 2½ ounces of sliced chicken. You may include a few olives, shredded carrots, and ½ sliced tomato or 5 grape tomatoes. Only 3 tablespoons of fat-free dressing, no bacon bits, no croutons.

BEVERAGES

- Choose one of the following:

Unlimited plain water (flat or fizzy)

1 cup of flavored water

1 cup of lemonade

1 cup of unsweetened iced tea

1 cup of juice (not from concentrate)

12-ounce can of diet soda (no more than 1 per day)

1 cup of low-fat, reduced-fat, or fat-free milk or unsweetened soy or almond milk

SNACK 4

- 1 SHRED POP popcorn *or* 1 cup of blueberries with 1 table-spoon of whipped cream *or* 2 medium kiwis *or* any other item 100 calories or less

Exercise

- **Amount of exercise today:** minimum 40 minutes. If you want to do more, all the better! Work as hard as you can! The key is to avoid doing steady-state exercise such as walking on the treadmill at the same speed and same incline for a period of time. Instead, try to vary your speed, your incline, the distances you cover. The goal here is to do high-intensity interval training.

- **Option 1:** Do the *SHRED 27 Burn* workout DVD.
- **Option 2:** Choose two of the cardiovascular exercises below, for a total of 40 minutes of exercise.

Walking/running outside or on treadmill

Jogging outside

Elliptical machine

Stationary or mobile bicycle

Swimming laps

Stair climber

200 jump rope revolutions

20-minute treadmill intervals

Zumba or other cardio dance workout

CHAPTER 6

Week 4: Tenacious

This is it! You have reached the homestretch of your four-week journey. Take a moment to acknowledge and appreciate the dedication that has brought you to this point. This has probably not been the easiest three weeks of your life, but hopefully you will have found the experience rewarding. Losing weight quickly but in a healthy manner requires you to get out of your comfort zone, something that you have likely done these last three weeks of your SUPER SHRED journey.

The definition of tenacious is "holding firmly, persistent, stubborn." That's why I have named this last week Tenacious. You must hold firm in your belief that you will continue to lose weight and progress ever closer to your goal, possibly even attain it. You must be persistent in the new, improved habits you have formed when it comes to eating, drinking, and exercising. Lastly, you must be *stubborn*. Despite all of the temptation to give up or slip off the plan, you will pursue your goals with vigor and stubbornness that simply won't let you quit. This week is about the final kick at the end of a long run when the finish line is within sight. You must remain steadfast so that all of what you've accomplished thus far will not be surrendered these last seven days. Instead, you will dig down, find your second wind, ignore the aches and fatigue, and burst across the finish line. Welcome to your last week of SUPER SHRED. Be nothing short of tenacious!

Please note that during this week the snack calories change between 100 to 150 depending on the day, so make sure you are paying attention. You can have a SHRED BAR or a bag of SHRED POP popcorn, any of the snacks listed in chapter 7, or other snacks that you find that meet the calorie requirements.

Week 4 will be easier than week 3, but it still requires you to work hard, especially since we're at the end. This week you will go back to four meals and you'll have one snack. (I can already see the smile on your face.) There is plenty of food to eat this week, so don't overdo it. And if you're not too hungry, simply leave something on your plate. Eat until you're satisfied, not stuffed. Last week should have taught you that you can make it with fewer calories. Below is a sample of what an eating schedule for this week might look like.

7:30 A.M.	8:30 A.M.	12:00 P.M.	1:30 P.M.	4:00 P.M.	7:30 P.M.
Awake	Meal 1	Meal 2	Snack	Meal 3	Meal 4

SUPER SHRED Week 4 Grocery List

This is a list that takes into consideration the different combinations of food and beverage items offered to you this week. Because the program has a lot of flexibility and choices, no one list can be constructed for everyone. In the list below you will find food and beverage opportunities. You can make the choices that fit your preferences and purchase accordingly. Note that there are some items that you *must* have. You should be sure to buy them so that you will have them on hand when the program calls for them. If you are a vegetarian, you don't need to eat the meat meals. Make appropriate substitutions, but be mindful of calorie counts.

FRUIT

- **Must:** 7 servings of fruit. This can be a combination of fruits such as berries, apples, bananas, pineapple, etc.
- **Optional:** 5 more servings of fresh fruit for low-fat yogurt and/or sides for sandwiches
- **Serving size:** 1 piece of fruit = 1 serving; ½ cup of berries = 1 serving

BREAKFAST OPTIONS

- 7 breakfast meals. Choose your combination from this list.

3 cups of oatmeal (1 cup cooked = 1 meal)

1 cup of Cream of Wheat or farina (1 cup cooked = 1 meal)

5 cups of sugar-free or low-sugar (under 5 grams) dry cereal (1 cup = 1 meal)

3 eggs

1 loaf of bread

1 pancake the size of a CD

1 strip of bacon (turkey or pork)

3 six-ounce containers of low-fat plain yogurt

2 grilled cheese sandwiches made with 2 slices of regular cheese on 2 pieces of 100 percent whole-grain or whole-wheat bread

BEVERAGES

- **Must:** 20 drink options for the week. Water is not included; you may have as much as you want. Choose your combinations from the list below. Then purchase your choices for the week.

18 cups of fresh juice

14 cups of coffee

7 twelve-ounce cans of diet soda

20 cups of low-fat, reduced-fat, or fat-free milk or unsweetened soy or almond milk

15 cups of unsweetened iced tea

12 cups of lemonade

15 cups of flavored water

SALADS

- **Must:** 3 large green garden salads, 1 medium green garden salad, 1 small green garden salad
- **Optional:** You will have other opportunities to have salads. Those opportunities are listed below. You should choose which of these you want, then purchase accordingly.

3 medium green garden salads

4 small green garden salads

VEGETABLES

- **Must:** 13 servings
- **Optional:** 4 servings. You will have other vegetable opportunities. If you choose them, purchase accordingly.
- **Serving size:** 1 serving is approximately the size of your fist

MEAT AND FISH

- **Must:** 3 servings. Choose from the list below. But note the maximum number of servings you may have for each option.
- **Optional:** 2 servings
- **Serving size:** 1 serving = 5 ounces, approximately the size of a deck and a half of playing cards, once cooked.
- Your maximum number of servings for the week will be 5 if you choose all of the optional servings. Make your choices from the list below, mixing them up. Remember, you must have at least 3 servings.

4 five-ounce pieces of chicken (skinless)

4 five-ounce pieces of turkey

5 five-ounce pieces of fish

SNACKS

- Choose 7 snacks for the entire week, such as nuts, Popsicles, chocolate-covered strawberries, and other items listed in chapter 7.

2 SHRED BARs or other snack items 150 calories or less

5 bags SHRED POP popcorn or other snack items 100 calories or less

SOUPS, SMOOTHIES, PROTEIN SHAKES

- **Must:** 9 servings from the items listed below. Each item must be 200 calories or less, with no added sugar. Choose the combination that you desire and purchase ingredients accordingly.

6 cups of low-salt soup (less than 480 milligrams sodium)

5 fruit smoothies

5 protein shakes

OPTIONAL MEAL CHOICES

- Throughout the week you will have the opportunity to have the meals listed below. Choose which of them you want, then purchase accordingly. You can choose all or none of them.

2 slices of small cheese pizza (no larger than 5 inches across the crust and 5 inches long)

1 serving of lasagna, with or without meat, 4 inches × 3 inches × 1 inch

2 veggie burgers (3 inches in diameter, ½ inch thick)

EXTRAS

- These are things you might want to have during the week, so stock up on them.

Salad toppings

Fat-free dressing for salad

Extra milk for cereal and coffee

Tomatoes

Lettuce

Cheese for sandwiches

Half-and-half

Buns for veggie burgers

Diced vegetables for omelet

SUPER SHRED Week 4 Guidelines

- Weigh yourself in the morning the day you start week 4 and make sure you record it. You will weigh yourself only once a week, so even if you are tempted, stay off the scale. Your body naturally fluctuates a couple of pounds from day to day. Measuring yourself every day could give you an inaccurate weight and unnecessarily stress you and lead you to believe you're not succeeding. Make sure you weigh yourself in the same manner each time: if you weighed in wearing certain clothes or no clothes at all, make sure you do the same this time around and as close to the same time of the day. Make sure you use the same scale each time, as different scales can be off by several pounds, thus destroying the accuracy of your measure.

• Do not skip meals. Even if you're not hungry, just have something during the allotted time. You can always grab a piece of fruit or something small during your mealtime. Also, you don't have to eat all of the meal. You can eat just some of it. If you're not hungry, don't stuff yourself. Just eat a little. The key is to eat at regularly scheduled times so that your body grows accustomed to these eating times. Each week will change, so it's important to quickly adapt to the week that you're in and its related schedule. During the course of the week you should never go more than 4 hours without eating something. Your meals should be 3 to 4 hours apart. Your snacks should fall about 1½ hours after meals. If you miss a meal or snack, you can't save it and eat it later or combine them. Once that time has passed, move on and hit your next mark.

• All of your shakes and smoothies this week must be 200 calories or less, with no added sugar. If you follow the recipes in the back of the book, they will fit this description. If you buy them from a store, be sure of the calorie count. Also, be mindful of the serving sizes of the drinks. If the recipe makes more than one serving, be sure you drink only one at that time. If the store-bought product contains more than 1 serving, just drink the equivalent of 1 serving and refrigerate the rest for next time.

- Snacks are optional, but highly recommended. The SHRED BARs and SHRED POP popcorn are suggested for many of your snacks, as they are specifically made with all of the nutritional guidelines in mind. However, you may have other snacks as long as they fall under the proper calorie count.

- Soups are an option, including store-bought soups. But make sure you look at the sodium content: no more than 480 milligrams *per serving.* Be mindful of the serving size. For the purpose of this plan, 1 serving is equivalent to 1 cup, whether you eat store-bought soup or make it fresh. You may have 1 saltine cracker with your soup.

- Consume 1 cup of water before *every* meal.

- You are allowed 2 cups of coffee each day, 1 cup at breakfast. Stay away from all those fancy coffee preparations—lattes, Frappuccinos, coffees that pile on the calories. A tablespoon of sugar and a little half-and-half or milk won't hurt, but don't go overboard.

- Canned and frozen fruits and vegetables are allowed. Please be aware of added ingredients. Make sure they are either packed in water or labeled "no sugar added." The key is to have food in its most natural state with the least amount of processing. Make sure you check the sodium levels, as they can be quite high: try to keep the amount to 480 milligrams of salt for any serving of food.

- While fresh-squeezed juice is definitely preferred, you can drink store-bought juice. Just make sure it says "not from concentrate" and "no sugar added." If you're a diabetic or have trouble regulating your blood sugar, choose a different beverage option, such as water, milk, or tea.

- The program doesn't spell out alcohol choices in the beverage section, but you are allowed to have a total of 3 alcoholic drinks for the week: 2 mixed drinks *or* 3 light beers *or* 3 glasses of wine *or* a combination of these drinks. Note serving sizes: 1 beer = 12 fluid ounces; 1 serving of wine = 5 fluid ounces (a little more than half a cup); a mixed drink has about 1½ fluid ounces of hard liquor. Also, you can't have them all in one day, so there's no saving them up for a big hit during the weekend. Liquid calories are stealthy and count just as much as food calories! And they definitely cause weight gain!

• You are allowed 1 diet soda per day if you desire. Regular soda is not recommended.

• Do not eat your last meal within 90 minutes of going to sleep. If because of circumstances you're eating late and know you're going right to bed, then consume half the meal.

• Spices are unlimited, so enjoy. Salt is not a spice. You are allowed to add no more than ½ teaspoon of salt to your food each day.

• If you are a vegetarian or diabetic or need to avoid certain foods owing to other medical conditions, it is completely acceptable to make substitutions. But make smart substitutions and be mindful of the portion sizes.

• Serving sizes: A 5-ounce serving of fish or meat after being cooked is typically the size of a deck and a half of playing cards. A serving of vegetables is typically the size of an adult's fist. A serving size of hot cereal is 1 cup of *cooked* cereal.

• You may have ½ pat of butter (about ½ teaspoon) with hot cereal.

• You may have 1 teaspoon of sugar (white or brown) or ½ teaspoon of honey with hot or cold cereals.

• If you must switch days or meals within a day for scheduling reasons, try to do so as infrequently as possible.

• If you need to rearrange your exercise regimen for scheduling reasons, it is permissible to do so.

SUPER SHRED WEEK 4, DAY 1

MEAL 1

- 1 piece of fruit or ½ cup of berries
- Choose one of the following:

1 cup of sugar-free cereal with low-fat, reduced-fat, or fat-free milk or unsweetened soy or almond milk

1 cup of oatmeal

1 grilled cheese sandwich made with 2 slices of regular cheese on 2 slices of 100 percent whole-wheat or whole-grain bread (little butter or cooking spray allowed)

1 six-ounce container of low-fat or fat-free yogurt; add fresh fruit

BEVERAGES

- 1 cup of fresh juice (not from concentrate) *or* 1 cup of tea *or* 1 cup of coffee

MEAL 2

- 1 medium green garden salad (3 cups of greens). You may include a few olives, shredded carrots, a few slices of beets,

onions, and ½ sliced tomato or 5 grape tomatoes. Only
2 tablespoons of fat-free dressing, no bacon bits, no croutons.

BEVERAGES

- Choose one of the following:

Unlimited plain water (flat or fizzy)

1 cup of flavored water

1 cup of lemonade

1 cup of unsweetened iced tea

1 cup of juice (not from concentrate)

12-ounce can of diet soda (no more than 1 per day)

1 cup of low-fat, reduced-fat, or fat-free milk or unsweetened soy
or almond milk

SNACK

- ⅓ cup of canned red kidney beans *or* 1 medium tomato with
  pinch of salt *or* 1 cup of cherries *or* 1 SHRED BAR *or*
  1 SHRED POP popcorn *or* any other item 150 calories or less

MEAL 3

- 1 serving of veggies
- Choose one of the following. Your choice must be 200 calories
  or less; no sugar added.

1 protein shake

1 cup of soup (no potatoes, no heavy cream). Good choices are
chicken noodle, vegetable, lentil, chickpea, split pea, black bean,
tomato basil, minestrone. Always be careful of sodium content!

BEVERAGES

- Choose one of the following:

Unlimited plain water (flat or fizzy)

1 cup of flavored water

1 cup of lemonade

1 cup of unsweetened iced tea

1 cup of juice (not from concentrate)

12-ounce can of diet soda (no more than 1 per day)

1 cup of low-fat, reduced-fat, or fat-free milk or unsweetened soy or almond milk

MEAL 4

- 3 servings of vegetables (please remember what counts as a serving size and don't overdo it)
- 1 cup of rice (brown or white)

BEVERAGES

- Choose one of the following:

Unlimited plain water (flat or fizzy)

1 cup of flavored water

1 cup of lemonade

1 cup of unsweetened iced tea

1 cup of juice (not from concentrate)

12-ounce can of diet soda (no more than 1 per day)

1 cup of low-fat, reduced-fat, or fat-free milk or unsweetened soy or almond milk

Exercise

- **Amount of exercise today:** minimum 40 minutes. If you want to do more, all the better! Work as hard as you can! The key is to avoid doing steady-state exercise such as walking on the treadmill at the same speed and same incline for a period of time. Instead, try to vary your speed, your incline, the distances you cover. The goal here is to do high-intensity interval training.
- **Option 1:** Do the *SHRED 27 Burn* workout DVD.
- **Option 2:** Choose two of the cardiovascular exercises below, for a total of 40 minutes of exercise.

Walking/running outside or on treadmill

Jogging outside

Elliptical machine

Stationary or mobile bicycle

Swimming laps

Stair climber

200 jump rope revolutions

20-minute treadmill intervals

Zumba or other cardio dance workout

SUPER SHRED WEEK 4, DAY 2

YOU'VE CONQUERED BIGGER ODDS! YOU'VE OVERCOME GREATER OBSTACLES! YOU'VE MADE A COMMITMENT TO BE A SUPER SHREDDER!!

MEAL I

- 1 piece of fruit or ½ cup of mixed berries
- Choose 1 of the following. Your choice must be 200 calories or less; no sugar added.

1 fruit smoothie

1 cup of soup (no potatoes, no heavy cream). Good choices are chicken noodle, vegetable, lentil, chickpea, split pea, black bean, tomato basil, minestrone. Always be careful of sodium content!

BEVERAGES

- Choose one of the following:

1 cup of fresh juice (not from concentrate)

1 cup of tea

1 cup of coffee

1 cup of low-fat, reduced-fat, or fat-free milk or unsweetened soy or almond milk

MEAL 2

- Choose one of the following:

1 chicken sandwich *or* 1 turkey sandwich (1 ounce of sliced meat) on 100 percent whole-grain or whole-wheat bread with a teaspoon of mustard or mayo, a slice of tomato, lettuce, and 1 slice of cheese. With your sandwich you may have a piece of fruit or a small green garden salad (2 cups of greens that can include a couple of olives, shredded carrots, a couple of small slices of tomato; only 1 tablespoon of fat-free dressing, no bacon bits, no croutons).

1 medium green garden salad (3 cups of greens). You may include a few olives, shredded carrots, a few slices of beets, onions, and ½ sliced tomato or 5 grape tomatoes. Only 2 tablespoons of fat-free dressing, no bacon bits, no croutons.

BEVERAGES

- Choose one of the following:

Unlimited plain water (flat or fizzy)

1 cup of flavored water

1 cup of lemonade

1 cup of unsweetened iced tea

1 cup of juice (not from concentrate)

12-ounce can of diet soda (no more than 1 per day)

1 cup of low-fat, reduced-fat, or fat-free milk or unsweetened soy or almond milk

Optional: 1 SHRED BAR *or* 1 SHRED POP popcorn *or* a 150-calorie snack

SNACK

- ⅓ cup of cooked quinoa *or* ¼ cup of low-fat granola *or* 1 SHRED POP popcorn *or* another 100-calorie snack

MEAL 3

- Choose one of the following:

1 veggie burger on a bun (whole-grain or whole-wheat preferred)

2 servings of vegetables and ½ cup of brown or white rice

5-ounce piece of fish (baked or grilled, not fried)

BEVERAGES

- Choose one of the following. Try to choose a different beverage from the one you chose in meal 2.

Unlimited plain water (flat or fizzy)

1 cup of flavored water

1 cup of lemonade

1 cup of unsweetened iced tea

1 cup of juice (not from concentrate)

12-ounce can of diet soda (no more than 1 per day)

1 cup of low-fat, reduced-fat, or fat-free milk or unsweetened soy or almond milk

MEAL 4

- 1 large green garden salad (4 cups of greens). You may include a few olives, shredded carrots, a few slices of beets, onions, and ½ sliced tomato or 5 grape tomatoes. Only 3 tablespoons of fat-free dressing, no bacon bits, no croutons.

BEVERAGES

- Choose one of the following. Try to choose a different beverage from the ones you chose in meals 2 and 3.

Unlimited plain water (flat or fizzy)

1 cup of flavored water

1 cup of lemonade

1 cup of unsweetened iced tea

1 cup of juice (not from concentrate)

12-ounce can of diet soda (no more than 1 per day)

1 cup of low-fat, reduced-fat, or fat-free milk or unsweetened soy or almond milk

Exercise

- **Amount of exercise today:** minimum 40 minutes. If you want to do more, all the better! Work as hard as you can! The key is to avoid doing steady state exercise such as walking on the treadmill at the same speed and same incline for a period of time. Instead, try to vary your speed, your incline, the distances you cover. The goal here is to do high-intensity interval training.
- **Option 1:** Do the *SHRED 27 Burn* workout.
- **Option 2:** Choose two of the cardiovascular exercises below, for a total of 40 minutes of exercise.

Walking/running outside or on treadmill

Jogging outside

Elliptical machine

Stationary or mobile bicycle

Swimming laps

Stair climber

200 jump rope revolutions

20-minute treadmill intervals

Zumba or other cardio dance workout

SUPER SHRED WEEK 4, DAY 3

YOU'VE CONQUERED BIGGER ODDS! YOU'VE OVERCOME GREATER OBSTACLES! YOU'VE MADE A COMMITMENT TO BE A SUPER SHREDDER!!

MEAL 1
- 1 piece of fruit or ½ cup of mixed berries
- Choose one of the following:

1 piece of 100 percent whole-grain or 100 percent whole-wheat toast and 1 hard-boiled egg

1 six-ounce container of low-fat or fat-free yogurt; add fresh fruit

1 cup of sugar-free cereal with low-fat, reduced-fat, or fat-free milk or unsweetened soy or almond milk

BEVERAGES
- Choose one of the following:

1 cup of fresh juice (not from concentrate)

1 cup of tea

1 cup of coffee

1 cup of milk (low-fat, reduced-fat, fat-free, soy, or almond)

MEAL 2

- Choose one of the following:

1 medium green garden salad (3 cups of greens). You may include a few olives, shredded carrots, a few slices of beets, onions, and ½ sliced tomato or 5 grape tomatoes. Only 2 tablespoons of fat-free dressing, no bacon bits, no croutons.

1 cup of soup (no potatoes, no heavy cream). Good choices are chicken noodle, vegetable, lentil, chickpea, split pea, black bean, tomato basil, minestrone. Always be careful of sodium content!

BEVERAGES

- Choose one of the following:

Unlimited plain water (flat or fizzy)

1 cup of flavored water

1 cup of lemonade

1 cup of unsweetened iced tea

1 cup of juice (not from concentrate)

12-ounce can of diet soda (no more than 1 per day)

1 cup of low-fat, reduced-fat, or fat-free milk or unsweetened soy or almond milk

SNACK

- 1 SHRED BAR *or* ½ cup of cottage cheese with 1 tablespoon of peanut butter mixed in *or* 2 tablespoons of low-fat hummus spread on crackers *or* any other item 150 calories or less

MEAL 3

- Choose one of the following. Your choice must not exceed 200 calories; no sugar added.

1 protein shake

1 fruit smoothie

1 cup of soup (no potatoes, no heavy cream). Good choices are chicken noodle, vegetable, lentil, chickpea, split pea, black bean, tomato basil, minestrone. Always be careful of sodium content!

BEVERAGES

- Choose one of the following. Try to choose a different beverage from the one you chose in meal 2.

Unlimited plain water (flat or fizzy)

1 cup of flavored water

1 cup of lemonade

1 cup of unsweetened iced tea

1 cup of juice (not from concentrate)

12-ounce can of diet soda (no more than 1 per day)

1 cup of low-fat, reduced-fat, or fat-free milk or unsweetened soy or almond milk

MEAL 4

- Choose one of the following:

2 slices of small cheese pizza (no larger than 5 inches across the crust and 5 inches long)

1 serving of lasagna, with or without meat, 4 inches × 3 inches × 1 inch

1 veggie burger (3 inches in diameter, ½ inch thick)

1 medium green garden salad (3 cups of greens). You may include a few olives, shredded carrots, a few slices of beets, onions, and ½ sliced tomato or 5 grape tomatoes. Only 2 tablespoons of fat-free dressing, no bacon bits, no croutons.

BEVERAGES

- Choose one of the following. Try to choose a different beverage from the ones you chose in meals 2 and 3.

Unlimited plain water (flat or fizzy)

1 cup of flavored water

1 cup of lemonade

1 cup of unsweetened iced tea

1 cup of juice (not from concentrate)

12-ounce can of diet soda (no more than 1 per day)

1 cup of low-fat, reduced-fat, or fat-free milk or unsweetened soy or almond milk

Exercise

- **Amount of exercise today:** minimum 60 minutes. If you want to do more, all the better! Work as hard as you can! The key is to avoid doing steady-state exercise such as walking on the treadmill at the same speed and same incline for a period of time. Instead, try to vary your speed, your incline, the distances you cover. The goal here is to do high-intensity interval training.
- **Option 1:** Do the *SHRED 27 Burn* workout DVD twice. Do this in two separate sessions at least 4 hours apart.

- **Option 2:** Choose two of the cardiovascular exercises below, for a total of 60 minutes of exercise. You can do this in two separate sessions.

Walking/running outside or on treadmill

Jogging outside

Elliptical machine

Stationary or mobile bicycle

Swimming laps

Stair climber

200 jump rope revolutions

20-minute treadmill intervals

Zumba or other cardio dance workout

SUPER SHRED WEEK 4, DAY 4
SUPER SHREDDER DAY!

YOU'VE CONQUERED BIGGER ODDS! YOU'VE OVERCOME GREATER OBSTACLES! YOU'VE MADE A COMMITMENT TO BE A SUPER SHREDDER!!

MEAL I

- 1 piece of fruit or ½ cup of mixed berries
- Choose one of the following. Your choice must be 200 calories or less; no sugar added.

1 protein shake

1 fruit smoothie

BEVERAGES

- Choose one of the following:

1 cup of tea

1 cup of coffee

1 cup of milk (low-fat, reduced-fat, fat-free, soy, or almond)

Unlimited plain water

MEAL 2

- 1 small green garden salad (2 cups of greens) that can include a couple of olives, shredded carrots, a couple of small slices of tomato. Only 1 tablespoon of fat-free dressing, no bacon bits or croutons.

BEVERAGES

- Choose one of the following:

Unlimited plain water (flat or fizzy)

1 cup of flavored water

1 cup of unsweetened iced tea

12-ounce can of diet soda (no more than 1 per day)

1 cup of low-fat, reduced-fat, or fat-free milk or unsweetened soy or almond milk

SNACK I

- 1 cup of grape tomatoes and 6 wheat crackers *or* 1 scoop of frozen yogurt *or* 1 SHRED POP popcorn *or* another 100-calorie snack

MEAL 3

- 2 servings of vegetables
- 1 cup of rice (brown or white)

BEVERAGES

- Choose one of the following. Try to choose a different beverage from the one you chose in meal 2.

Unlimited plain water (flat or fizzy)

1 cup of flavored water

1 cup of unsweetened iced tea

12-ounce can of diet soda (no more than 1 per day)

1 cup of low-fat, reduced-fat, or fat-free milk or unsweetened soy or almond milk

MEAL 4

- 1 cup of soup (no potatoes, no heavy cream). Good choices are chicken noodle, vegetable, lentil, chickpea, split pea, black bean, tomato basil, minestrone. Always be careful of sodium content!

BEVERAGES

- Choose one of the following. Try to choose a different beverage from the ones you chose in meals 2 and 3.

Unlimited plain water (flat or fizzy)

1 cup of flavored water

1 cup of unsweetened iced tea

12-ounce can of diet soda (no more than 1 per day)

Exercise

- **Amount of exercise today:** minimum 30 minutes. If you want to do more, all the better! Work as hard as you can! The key is to avoid doing steady-state exercise such as walking on the treadmill at the same speed and same incline for a period of time. Instead, try to vary your speed, your incline, the distances you cover. The goal here is to do high-intensity interval training.
- **Option 1:** Do the *SHRED 27 Burn* workout DVD.
- **Option 2:** Choose two of the cardiovascular exercises below, for a total of 30 minutes of exercise.

Walking/running outside or on treadmill

Jogging outside

Elliptical machine

Stationary or mobile bicycle

Swimming laps

Stair climber

200 jump rope revolutions

20-minute treadmill intervals

Zumba or other cardio dance workout

SUPER SHRED WEEK 4, DAY 5

MEAL I

- 1 piece of fruit or ½ cup of mixed berries
- Choose one of the following:

1 pancake the size of a CD with 1 slice of bacon (turkey or pork)

1 grilled cheese sandwich made with 2 slices of regular cheese on 2 slices of 100 percent whole-wheat or 100 percent whole-grain bread (little butter or cooking spray allowed)

1 cup of sugar-free cereal with low-fat, reduced-fat, or fat-free milk or unsweetened soy or almond milk

1 six-ounce container of low-fat or fat-free yogurt; add fresh fruit

BEVERAGES

- Choose one of the following:

1 cup of fresh juice (not from concentrate)

1 cup of tea

1 cup of coffee

1 cup of milk (low-fat, reduced-fat, fat-free, soy, or almond)

Unlimited plain water

MEAL 2

- Choose one of the following. Your choice must not exceed 200 calories; no sugar added.

1 protein shake

1 fruit smoothie

BEVERAGES

- Choose one of the following:

Unlimited plain water (flat or fizzy)

1 cup of flavored water

1 cup of lemonade

1 cup of unsweetened iced tea

1 cup of juice (not from concentrate)

12-ounce can of diet soda (no more than 1 per day)

1 cup of low-fat, reduced-fat, or fat-free milk or unsweetened soy or almond milk

SNACK

- 1 SHRED POP popcorn *or* 1 SHRED BAR *or* any other item 150 calories or less

MEAL 3

- 1 large green garden salad (4 cups of greens). You may include a few olives, shredded carrots, a few slices of beets, onions, and ½ sliced tomato or 5 grape tomatoes. Only 3 tablespoons of fat-free dressing, no bacon bits, no croutons.

BEVERAGES

- Choose one of the following. Try to choose a different beverage from the one you chose in meal 2.

Unlimited plain water (flat or fizzy)

1 cup of flavored water

1 cup of lemonade

1 cup of unsweetened iced tea

1 cup of juice (not from concentrate)

12-ounce can of diet soda (no more than 1 per day)

1 cup of low-fat, reduced-fat, or fat-free milk or unsweetened soy or almond milk

MEAL 4

- 2 servings of vegetables
- Choose one of the following:

5-ounce piece of chicken (baked or grilled, not fried, no skin)

5-ounce piece of turkey (not fried, no skin)

5-ounce piece of fish (baked or grilled, not fried)

BEVERAGES

- Choose one of the following. Try to choose a different beverage from the ones you chose in meals 2 and 3.

Unlimited plain water (flat or fizzy)

1 cup of flavored water

1 cup of lemonade

1 cup of unsweetened iced tea

1 cup of juice (not from concentrate)

12-ounce can of diet soda (no more than 1 per day)

1 cup of low-fat, reduced-fat, or fat-free milk or unsweetened soy or almond milk

Exercise

- Rest Day! This is a rest day, especially if you are aching and your muscles need recovery. But if you feel up to it and you decide to do some exercise on your own, that is completely allowed. Thirty minutes of cardio training will always serve you well, so feel free to get in some extra work. Each exercise session will move you closer to your goal!

SUPER SHRED WEEK 4, DAY 6

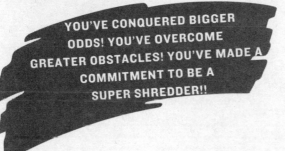

YOU'VE CONQUERED BIGGER ODDS! YOU'VE OVERCOME GREATER OBSTACLES! YOU'VE MADE A COMMITMENT TO BE A SUPER SHREDDER!!

MEAL 1
- 1 piece of fruit or ½ cup of mixed berries
- Choose one of the following:

1 cup of oatmeal

1 cup of Cream of Wheat or farina

1 cup of sugar-free cereal with low-fat, reduced-fat, or fat-free milk or unsweetened soy or almond milk

BEVERAGES

- Choose one of the following:

1 cup of fresh juice (not from concentrate)

1 cup of tea

1 cup of coffee

1 cup of milk (low-fat, reduced-fat, fat-free, soy, or almond)

MEAL 2

- 1 cup of soup (no potatoes, no heavy cream). Good choices
  are chicken noodle, vegetable, lentil, chickpea, split pea,
  black bean, tomato basil, minestrone. Always be careful of
  sodium content!
- 1 serving of vegetables

BEVERAGES

- Choose one of the following:

Unlimited plain water (flat or fizzy)

1 cup of flavored water

1 cup of lemonade

1 cup of unsweetened iced tea

1 cup of juice (not from concentrate)

12-ounce can of diet soda (no more than 1 per day)

1 cup of low-fat, reduced-fat, or fat-free milk or unsweetened soy
or almond milk

SNACK

- 2 celery stalks with 2 tablespoons of natural peanut butter *or* ¼ cup of yogurt-covered raisins *or* 1 SHRED BAR *or* another snack item 150 calories or less

MEAL 3

- Choose one of the following:

1 chicken sandwich (1 ounce sliced meat) on 100 percent whole-grain or whole-wheat bread with 1 teaspoon of mustard or mayo, 1 slice of tomato, lettuce, and 1 slice of cheese. With your sandwich you can have a piece of fruit or a small green garden salad (2 cups of greens) that can include a couple of olives, shredded carrots, a couple of small slices of tomato. Only 1 tablespoon of fat-free dressing, no bacon bits or croutons.

1 turkey sandwich (1 ounce sliced meat) on 100 percent whole-grain or whole-wheat bread with 1 teaspoon of mustard or mayo, 1 slice of tomato, lettuce, and 1 slice of cheese. With your sandwich you can have a piece of fruit or a small green garden salad (2 cups of greens) that can include a couple of olives, shredded carrots, a couple of small slices of tomato. Only 1 tablespoon of fat-free dressing, no bacon bits or croutons.

2 servings of vegetables and ½ cup of brown rice

BEVERAGES

- Choose one of the following. Try to choose a different beverage from the one you chose in meal 2.

Unlimited plain water (flat or fizzy)

1 cup of flavored water

1 cup of lemonade

1 cup of unsweetened iced tea

1 cup of juice (not from concentrate)

12-ounce can of diet soda (no more than 1 per day)

1 cup of low-fat, reduced-fat, or fat-free milk or unsweetened soy or almond milk

MEAL 4
- 3 servings of vegetables
- 1 cup of brown or white rice

BEVERAGES
- Choose one of the following. Try to choose a different beverage from the ones you chose in meals 2 and 3.

Unlimited plain water (flat or fizzy)

1 cup of flavored water

1 cup of lemonade

1 cup of unsweetened iced tea

1 cup of juice (not from concentrate)

12-ounce can of diet soda (no more than 1 per day)

1 cup of low-fat, reduced-fat, or fat-free milk or unsweetened soy or almond milk

Exercise

- **Amount of exercise today:** minimum 60 minutes. If you want to do more, all the better! Work as hard as you can! The key is to avoid doing steady-state exercise such as walking on the treadmill at the same speed and same incline for a period of time. Instead, try to vary your speed, your incline, the distances you cover. The goal here is to do high-intensity interval training.

- **Option 1:** Do the *SHRED 27 Burn* workout DVD twice. Do this in two separate sessions at least 4 hours apart.
- **Option 2:** Choose two of the cardiovascular exercises below, for a total of 60 minutes of exercise. You can do this in two separate sessions.

Walking/running outside or on treadmill

Jogging outside

Elliptical machine

Stationary or mobile bicycle

Swimming laps

Stair climber

200 jump rope revolutions

20-minute treadmill intervals

Zumba or other cardio dance workout

SUPER SHRED WEEK 4, DAY 7

YOU'VE CONQUERED BIGGER ODDS! YOU'VE OVERCOME GREATER OBSTACLES! YOU'VE MADE A COMMITMENT TO BE A SUPER SHREDDER!!

MEAL I

- 1 piece of fruit or ½ cup of mixed berries
- Choose one of the following:

1 cup of oatmeal

1 cup of sugar-free cereal with low-fat, reduced-fat, or fat-free milk or unsweetened soy or almond milk

2 egg whites or 1 egg-white omelet with diced veggies

Optional: 1 piece of 100 percent whole-grain or whole-wheat toast (½ pat butter or ½ teaspoon jelly)

BEVERAGES

- Choose one of the following:

1 cup of fresh juice (not from concentrate)

1 cup of tea

1 cup of coffee

1 cup of milk (low-fat, reduced-fat, fat-free, soy, or almond)

MEAL 2

- Choose one of the following. Your choice must not exceed 200 calories; no sugar added.

1 protein shake

1 fruit smoothie

1 cup of soup (no potatoes, no heavy cream). Good choices are chicken noodle, vegetable, lentil, chickpea, split pea, black bean, tomato basil, minestrone. Always be careful of sodium content!

BEVERAGES

- Choose one of the following:

Unlimited plain water (flat or fizzy)

1 cup of flavored water

1 cup of unsweetened iced tea

12-ounce can of diet soda (no more than 1 per day)

1 cup of low-fat, reduced-fat, or fat-free milk or unsweetened soy or almond milk

SNACK

- 1 piece of fruit *or* 2 tablespoons of black bean salsa spread over 3 two-inch slices of eggplant *or* 1 SHRED POP popcorn *or* another 100-calorie snack

MEAL 3

- 1 serving of vegetables
- Choose from one of the following:

5-ounce piece of chicken (no skin, baked or grilled, not fried)

5-ounce piece of turkey (no skin, not fried)

5-ounce piece of fish (baked or grilled, not fried)

BEVERAGES

- Choose one of the following. Try to choose a different beverage from the one you chose in meal 2.

Unlimited plain water (flat or fizzy)

1 cup of flavored water

1 cup of unsweetened iced tea

12-ounce can of diet soda (no more than 1 per day)

1 cup of low-fat, reduced-fat, or fat-free milk or unsweetened soy or almond milk

MEAL 4

- 1 large green garden salad (4 cups of greens). You may include a few olives, shredded carrots, a few slices of beets, onions, and ½ sliced tomato or 5 grape tomatoes. Only 3 tablespoons of fat-free dressing, no bacon bits, no croutons.

BEVERAGES

- Choose one of the following. Try to choose a different beverage from the ones you chose in meals 2 and 3.

Unlimited plain water (flat or fizzy)

1 cup of flavored water

1 cup of lemonade

1 cup of unsweetened iced tea

1 cup of juice (not from concentrate)

12-ounce can of diet soda (no more than 1 per day)

1 cup of low-fat, reduced-fat, or fat-free milk or unsweetened soy
or almond milk

Exercise

- **Amount of exercise today:** minimum 40 minutes. If you want
  to do more, all the better! Work as hard as you can! The key is
  to avoid doing steady-state exercise such as walking on the
  treadmill at the same speed and same incline for a period of
  time. Instead, try to vary your speed, your incline, the distances you cover. The goal here is to do high-intensity interval
  training.
- **Option 1:** Do the *SHRED 27 Burn* workout DVD.
- **Option 2:** Choose two of the cardiovascular exercises below,
  for a total of 40 minutes of exercise.

Walking/running outside or on treadmill

Jogging outside

Elliptical machine

Stationary or mobile bicycle

Swimming laps

Stair climber

200 jump rope revolutions

20-minute treadmill intervals

Zumba or other cardio dance workout

[CHAPTER 7]

SUPER SHRED Snacks

Snacking is an important part of the SUPER SHRED strategy. One of the biggest mistakes people make when trying to lose weight is in their distribution of meals and snacks. Allowing too much time to lapse between meals can be counterproductive to your efforts, because having intense hunger when you finally sit down for a meal can lead to overeating and the consumption of too many calories. Proper snacking can avoid this and, in fact, encourage you to actually consume less at your meals, because your hunger isn't too intense.

Snacking can also keep your metabolism chugging along. Imagine your metabolism is a fireplace and logs are the equivalent of calories. The larger the fire, the more logs (calories) you burn. Snacking is the equivalent of stoking a fire. The more you do it at the right time and in the appropriate manner, the better and longer the fire will burn. Snacking stokes your metabolism, and this is important in our overall strategy of burning more calories.

The snacks during the daily meal plans are optional, but I strongly recommend that you make use of them. I have developed special SHRED BARs that are low in calories, gluten-free, low in carbohydrates, and high in fiber and other critical nutrients. You can always have a SHRED BAR for your 150-calorie snack. They are tasty, make you feel full, and fit perfectly in the plan. You can also have a bag of SHRED POP popcorn. There are a variety of flavors, such as white cheddar and barbecue, and I've made sure the ingredients are healthy and provide you with more nutritional benefits. The popcorn can be used for any of the snack times in the book. You can find out where to get these snacks by going to www.doctoriansmith.com.

If you want variety in your snacks, you have a treasure trove of options. This chapter is broken up into two snack lists—150 calories and 100 calories. This list is here for your convenience as you plan your week, but you can eat snacks that are not on the list as well, as long as they fall into the calorie specifications the meal plan calls for. Snacks can be extremely helpful when it comes to keeping your appetite in check, so if you decide to choose something not in the book, just make it a wise choice. Consuming sweets that have little or no nutritional value is a complete waste of an opportunity to suppress your hunger. Many sweets also deprive you of the opportunity to benefit from a quick dose of powerful nutrients. Snack well!

100-Calorie Snacks

- 1 package SHRED POP popcorn
- 1 cup of blueberries with 1 tablespoon whipped cream
- Citrus-berry salad: 1 cup mixed berry salad (raspberries, strawberries, blueberries, and blackberries) tossed with 1 tablespoon fresh-squeezed orange juice

- 2 medium kiwifruits
- Kale chips: ⅔ cup raw kale (stems removed) baked with 1 teaspoon olive oil at 400 degrees until crisp
- ½ medium baked potato, touch of butter
- 1 medium red pepper, sliced, with 2 tablespoons soft goat cheese
- 10 baby carrots with 2 tablespoons hummus
- White bean salad: ⅓ cup white beans, pinch of lemon juice, ¼ cup diced tomatoes, 4 cucumber slices
- ⅓ cup wasabi peas
- ⅕ avocado smashed on a whole-grain cracker, sprinkled with balsamic vinegar and sea salt
- Tropical cottage cheese: ½ cup nonfat cottage cheese with ½ cup chopped fresh mango and pineapple
- ½ cup fat-free yogurt and ½ cup blueberries
- Chickpea salad: ¼ cup chickpeas with 1 tablespoon chopped scallions, a squeeze of lemon juice, and ¼ cup diced tomatoes
- ½ whole-wheat English muffin topped with 1 teaspoon fruit butter
- Stuffed figs: 2 small dried figs stuffed with 1 tablespoon reduced-fat ricotta and sprinkled with cinnamon
- 2 stalks celery
- 1 cup lettuce drizzled with 2 tablespoons fat-free dressing
- 1 hard-boiled egg and ½ cup sugar snap peas
- ½ cup raisin bran
- Strawberry salad: 1 cup raw spinach with ½ cup sliced strawberries and 1 tablespoon balsamic vinegar
- 1 thin brown-rice cake spread with 1 tablespoon peanut butter
- Crunchy kale salad: 1 cup chopped kale leaves with 1 teaspoon honey and 1 tablespoon balsamic vinegar
- 1 medium cucumber

- ½ cup crabmeat, canned
- 1 cup grape tomatoes and 6 wheat crackers
- 3 ounces cod, cooked
- 1 nonfat mozzarella cheese stick with half of a medium-size apple (about the size of a baseball), skin left on and sliced
- 3 teaspoons natural peanut butter
- Greek tomatoes: 1 tomato (about the size of a tennis ball) chopped and mixed with 1 tablespoon feta and a squeeze of lemon juice
- 2 cups watermelon chunks
- 3 dried apricots stuffed with 1 tablespoon crumbled blue cheese
- ½ cup low-fat salsa and 5 small (bite-size) tortilla chips
- Turkey roll-ups: 4 slices smoked turkey rolled up and dipped in 2 teaspoons honey mustard
- ½ cup nonfat Greek yogurt with a dash of cinnamon and 1 teaspoon honey
- Cheesy breaded tomatoes: 2 roasted plum tomatoes sliced and topped with 2 tablespoons bread crumbs and a sprinkle of parmesan cheese
- 1 cup fresh red raspberries with 2 tablespoons plain yogurt
- 2 graham cracker squares and 1 teaspoon peanut butter, sprinkled with cinnamon
- 1 baked medium tomato sprinkled with 2 teaspoons parmesan cheese
- Small baked apple (about the size of a tennis ball) dusted with cinnamon
- Chocolate banana: ½ frozen banana dipped in two squares of melted dark chocolate
- Cucumber sandwich: ½ English muffin with 2 tablespoons cottage cheese and 3 slices cucumber

- 15 mini pretzel sticks with 2 tablespoons fat-free cream cheese
- 1 small scoop low-fat frozen yogurt
- Spicy black beans: ¼ cup black beans with 1 tablespoon salsa and 1 tablespoon nonfat Greek yogurt
- 11 blue-corn tortilla chips
- Cucumber salad: 1 large cucumber, sliced, with 2 tablespoons red onion and 2 tablespoons apple cider vinegar
- ⅓ cup cooked quinoa
- 2 pineapple rounds, each ¼ inch thick, grilled or sautéed
- 3 tablespoons all-natural granola
- ¼ cup low-fat granola
- 9 to 10 black olives
- 7 saltines
- 2 cups air-popped popcorn with 1 teaspoon butter
- 25 oyster crackers
- 1 large carrot, raw
- Watermelon salad: 1 cup raw spinach with ⅔ cup diced watermelon, sprinkled with 1 tablespoon balsamic vinegar
- 25 peanuts, oil-roasted
- 2 tablespoons flaxseeds
- 2 ounces salmon, fresh, cooked
- 1½ cups puffed rice
- 3 ounces tuna, canned in water
- 3 tablespoons roasted, unsalted soy nuts
- ½ cup diced cantaloupe topped with ½ cup low-fat cottage cheese
- ½ sheet matzo
- ⅔ ounce dark chocolate
- ¾ cup carrots, cooked
- 1 cup broccoli florets with 2 tablespoons dip

- 2 ounces mussels, cooked
- 4 mini rice cakes with 2 tablespoons low-fat cottage cheese
- 1 seven-grain Belgian waffle
- 1 strip of low-fat string cheese
- Black bean salsa over 3 eggplant slices
- ¾ ounce sharp cheddar cheese cubes
- 3 cups of air-popped popcorn
- 1 medium tomato sliced with a sprinkle of feta cheese and olive oil
- 3 to 4 tablespoons dried cherries
- 1 nectarine
- 1 fresh pomegranate
- ½ pound fruit salad
- 4 dates
- 3 figs, fresh
- ⅓ cup canned red kidney beans
- 7 animal crackers, plain
- About 40 Pepperidge Farm goldfish
- 1 medium tomato, raw, pinch of salt
- 2 ounces salmon, smoked
- 4 large sea scallops, cooked
- 6 oysters
- 2 tablespoons poppy seeds
- 2 tablespoons pumpkin seeds
- 6 dried apricots
- 3 crackers lightly spread with peanut butter
- 3 medium breadsticks with hummus
- 2 small peaches
- 1 cup strawberries
- 1 medium corn on the cob with seasoning
- 30 grapes

- ½ cup unsweetened applesauce with 1 slice whole-wheat toast, cut into 4 strips for dunking
- 4 to 6 ounces nonfat or low-fat yogurt
- 3 pineapple rings in natural juices
- 3 oven-baked potato wedges
- 1 rice cake with 1 tablespoon guacamole
- 1 cup radishes, sliced or chopped
- ½ cup oat cereal, toasted
- 6 large clams
- 3 ounces crabmeat, fresh, cooked
- 1½ ounces halibut, Pacific, wild-caught, fresh, cooked
- 2 ounces lobster, cooked
- 2 ounces bay scallops, cooked
- 2 ounces yellowfin tuna, fresh, cooked
- 17 pecans
- 2 ounces lean roast beef
- 1 can (11.5 ounces) low-sodium V8 100 percent vegetable juice
- Medium grapefruit sprinkled with ½ teaspoon sugar, broiled if desired
- Portobello mushroom stuffed with roast veggies and 1 teaspoon shredded low-fat cheese
- 8 small shrimps and 3 tablespoons cocktail sauce
- 1 tablespoon peanuts and 2 tablespoons dried cranberries
- 20 grapes with 15 peanuts
- 2 slices deli turkey breast
- 1 cup sliced zucchini, seasoned to taste
- 10 cashews
- 2 tablespoons sunflower seeds
- 1 cup cherries
- ½ cup clam chowder, preferably tomato-based

150-Calorie Snacks

- 1 SHRED BAR
- 4 saltine jelly sandwiches: sugar-free jelly between 2 saltine crackers; 8 crackers in all
- ½ cup low-fat cottage cheese with 1 tablespoon natural peanut butter mixed in
- 5 Ritz crackers smeared with a little peanut butter
- 1 packet plain instant oatmeal, ½ cup fresh blueberries, sprinkle of cinnamon
- 1 cup grape tomatoes
- 1 medium apple, sliced, with 1 tablespoon natural peanut butter spread on the slices
- ½ blueberry muffin
- 1 medium sliced red bell pepper with ¼ cup guacamole
- 1 Jell-O chocolate fudge sugar-free pudding with 5 slices strawberries and 1 tablespoon whipped cream
- 1½ cups fresh fruit salad
- 2 cups air-popped popcorn sprinkled with parmesan cheese
- ¼ cup yogurt-covered raisins
- 1½ cups frozen grapes
- 2 stalks celery and 2 tablespoons natural peanut butter
- Mediterranean salad: 1 tomato, 1 medium cucumber, ½ red onion, diced and sprinkled with 2 tablespoons low-fat feta cheese
- 1 cup sugar snap peas with 3 tablespoons low-fat hummus
- Watermelon treat: 1 cup diced watermelon topped with 2 tablespoons crumbled feta cheese
- ½ cup roasted chickpeas
- 1 large apple, sliced, sprinkled with cinnamon

- 1 slice Swiss cheese and 8 olives
- Tasty pepper: sliced bell pepper, marinated in 1 tablespoon balsamic vinegar, salt, and pepper
- 1 cup strawberries dipped in 1 tablespoon melted sweet chocolate chips
- 2 dill pickle spears
- 16 cashews
- Tuna salad: 1 can (5 ounces) light tuna in water, 1 tablespoon low-fat mayo, and 1 diced sweet pickle
- 1 cup of Cheerios
- 46 pistachios
- 2 Dole fruit juice bars
- 12 small baked tortilla chips and ½ cup salsa
- 2 medium-size nectarines
- 21 raw almonds
- 6 cucumber, cherry tomato, ball of mozzarella skewers
- Stuffed tomatoes: 10 halved grape tomatoes stuffed with a mixture of ¼ cup low-fat ricotta cheese, 1 tablespoon diced black olives, and a pinch of black pepper
- ¼ red bell pepper, sliced, ¼ cup thin carrot slices, ¼ cup guacamole
- ½ cup sugar-free applesauce mixed with 10 pecan halves
- 20 medium-size cherries
- 2 tablespoons hummus spread on 4 crackers
- 1 cup raspberries topped with 2 tablespoons whipped cream
- ½ cup black beans topped with 2 tablespoons guacamole
- 1½ strips low-fat string cheese
- ½ cup low-fat cottage cheese with ¼ cup fresh pineapple slices
- 1 packet instant oatmeal with fresh fruit sprinkled on top
- ½ cup roasted pumpkin seeds, lightly salted to taste

- 4 ounces chicken breast wrapped in lettuce and topped with dill mustard
- 2 ounces turkey jerky
- ½ avocado topped with diced tomatoes and a pinch of pepper
- ⅓ cup dried apricots
- 10 baked whole-wheat pita chips and 3 tablespoons salsa
- ½ cup shelled pistachios
- ½ cup natural apple chips (no sugar or preservatives added)
- 2 scoops sorbet
- 9 chocolate-covered almonds
- 1 cup grapes with 10 almonds
- Frozen banana slices
- Turkey-wrapped avocado: ¼ avocado sliced into strips and wrapped in 3 ounces deli turkey meat
- Chocolate-dipped pretzels: melt semisweet chocolate morsels in a microwave; dip 3 honey pretzel sticks in chocolate; put pretzels in freezer until chocolate sets
- Medium orange sliced and topped with 2 tablespoons chopped walnuts
- 1 small chocolate pudding
- 2 hard-boiled eggs with a pinch of salt and pepper
- 4 chocolate-chip cookies, each a little larger than the size of a poker chip
- Applesauce and cereal: 1 applesauce pouch and ½ cup dry cereal
- 50 Pepperidge Farm goldfish
- Hummus and cucumbers: cut up half a large cucumber and combine it with 2 tablespoons hummus
- 9 Ritz crackers
- ¾ cup halved strawberries topped with 3 tablespoons light whipped cream

- 16 saltines
- 1 Nestlé Crunch reduced-fat ice-cream bar
- 1 small banana, sliced, and ½ ounce dark chocolate
- ½ cup Breyers light natural vanilla ice cream
- 1 medium mango
- ½ peanut butter and jelly sandwich
- 2 frozen fruit bars
- ¾ cup steamed edamame (baby soybeans)
- 6 watermelon skewers: place 1 cube watermelon, 1 small cube feta cheese, and 1 slice cucumber on each of 6 toothpicks
- 2 Popsicles
- ½ cup roasted pumpkin seeds (keep in shells)
- 7 olives stuffed with 1 tablespoon blue cheese
- Brown-rice vegetable sushi rolls, 5 pieces
- 1 ounce pretzels and 1 teaspoon honey mustard
- 2 Fudgsicles
- Small baked potato topped with salsa
- 1 cup yogurt parfait and 1 tablespoon of granola
- 5 pitted dates stuffed with 5 whole almonds
- Blueberries and sorbet: ½ cup fruit sorbet topped with ½ cup blueberries
- 10 baby carrots dipped in 2 tablespoons light salad dressing
- Turkey wrap: 2 slices deli turkey breast, whole-grain flatbread, sliced tomatoes and cucumbers, and lettuce
- 25 frozen red seedless grapes
- ¾ cup roasted cauliflower, pinch of sea salt
- 4 pot stickers dipped in 2 teaspoons reduced-sodium soy sauce
- 6 dried figs
- Loaded pepper slices: 1 cup red bell pepper slices topped with ¼ cup warmed black beans and 1 tablespoon guacamole
- Kiwifruit and oats: slice of kiwifruit with ½ cup of oat cereal

- 8 Wheat Thins with Laughing Cow light cheese wedge
- 1 cup sugar snap peas with 3 tablespoons hummus
- 1 medium pear and 1 cup low-fat or fat-free milk
- Baby burrito: 6-inch corn tortilla, 2 tablespoons bean dip, and 2 tablespoons salsa
- 2 squares graham crackers and 8 ounces skim milk
- 1 medium papaya with a squeeze of lime juice on top; sprinkle of chili powder optional
- Peanut butter and jelly: ½ whole-grain English muffin, 1 tablespoon peanut butter, and no-sugar-added jelly
- 10 walnut halves and 1 sliced kiwifruit
- English muffin pizza: top whole-wheat English muffin with 1 tablespoon of tomato sauce and 1 tablespoon parmesan cheese, and broil
- Egg salad sandwich: ½ hard-boiled egg, ½ teaspoon low-fat mayo, and spices spread on half of a toasted whole-wheat or whole-grain bagel
- Cottage cheese and almond butter: ½ cup no-salt-added 1 percent cottage cheese mixed with 1 tablespoon almond butter
- 1 small baked potato topped with a mixture of salsa and 1 tablespoon of low-fat cheddar cheese
- 1 can of tuna, drained, seasoned to taste
- ½ medium avocado sprinkled with sea salt
- 1 Skinny Cow ice-cream sandwich
- 4 turkey slices and 1 medium apple, sliced

[CHAPTER 8]

SUPER SHRED Smoothies

These smoothie recipes are specifically designed to be simple, tasty, and convenient. Please make sure that you pay attention to the serving size for each recipe. If there are multiple servings for a recipe, it's important that you don't consume all of it at once. Store the extra servings and consume at a later time. You can modify the recipes as they fit your taste, but be careful not to add ingredients that are going to increase the calorie count. You can, however, make smart substitutions. Switching blackberries for blueberries or apples for pears is completely acceptable. Just remember, adding other ingredients such as honey, milk, and sugar will increase your calorie count, so do so on a limited basis.

There are different ways to prepare the fruits in smoothies. Obviously, using fresh fruit is most desirable, as it delivers the nutrients in their most natural, unaltered state to the blender. But be mindful of the possibility and convenience of frozen fruits. Make sure you choose frozen fruits in packaging that says "no added sugar." There are natural carbohydrates and sugars in all fruits; these will be listed in the nutrition facts on the back of the package. Don't be put off by these numbers in your frozen fruits. Both sugar count and total carbohydrate count are important, but for our purposes, the total carbohydrate number is what you should pay attention to when reviewing the nutrition facts. In general, you want to keep the total carbohydrate number to less than 20 grams.

• MANGO MADNESS •

¼ cup mango cubes, fresh or frozen

⅓ cup mango juice

¼ cup mashed avocado

¼ cup fat-free vanilla yogurt

2 teaspoons freshly squeezed
  lime juice

2 teaspoons sugar

7 ice cubes

Combine the mango, mango juice, avocado, yogurt, lime juice, sugar, and ice cubes in a blender. Process until smooth.

• CUCUMBER-PEAR VITALIZER •

TOTAL TIME: 5 MINUTES

SERVINGS: 1

UNDER 200 CALORIES

1 small cucumber, peeled and seeded

½ medium green pear, peeled and cored

Pinch of ground ginger

6 ice cubes

Slice the cucumber into quarters. Blend cucumber with 1 tablespoon of water. Add pear, ginger, and ice to cucumber purée and blend on high.

• WATERMELON SPRITZ •

TOTAL TIME: 5 MINUTES

SERVINGS: 1

UNDER 200 CALORIES

2½ cups seedless watermelon

⅓ cup fat-free yogurt

1 tablespoon fresh mint

1 teaspoon sugar (optional)

6 ice cubes

Combine all ingredients in a blender and purée until smooth.

• THE CHOCOLATE RAZZY •

TOTAL TIME: 5 MINUTES

SERVINGS: 1

UNDER 200 CALORIES

1 cup fresh or frozen raspberries

4 tablespoons fat-free vanilla yogurt

¼ cup chocolate chips

⅓ cup fat-free or low-fat milk

3 ice cubes

Combine all ingredients in a blender and purée until smooth.

• THE PURPLE MASH •

TOTAL TIME: 5 MINUTES

SERVINGS: 2

UNDER 200 CALORIES

1 cup fresh or frozen blueberries

½ cup fresh or frozen pineapple
   chunks

½ cup fat-free vanilla yogurt

⅓ cup low-fat vanilla soy milk

1 tablespoon lemon juice

2 teaspoons honey or sugar (optional)

Combine the blueberries and pineapple and blend. Add the rest of the ingredients and purée until smooth. This recipe makes multiple servings; drink only one at this time.

• THE GREAT BLUE PINE •

TOTAL TIME: 5 MINUTES

SERVINGS: 2

UNDER 200 CALORIES

1 cup fresh or frozen blueberries

1 medium banana, peeled and sliced

¼ cup chopped fresh pineapple

1½ cups fresh baby spinach

⅓ cup orange juice

⅓ cup frozen dark cherries

½ cup fat-free vanilla yogurt

Combine all ingredients in a blender and purée until smooth. This recipe makes multiple servings; drink only one at this time.

• LEMON ORANGE ELIXIR •

TOTAL TIME: 5 MINUTES

SERVINGS: 1

UNDER 200 CALORIES

4 tablespoons fat-free or low-fat lemon yogurt

1 medium orange, peeled, sliced into sections, and seeded

⅔ cups fat-free milk or unsweetened soy milk

8 ice cubes

2 teaspoons flaxseed oil (optional)

Combine all ingredients in a blender and purée until smooth.

• THE DOWN UNDER SPECTACULAR •

TOTAL TIME: 5 MINUTES

SERVINGS: 3

UNDER 200 CALORIES

2 cups cubed honeydew

1 kiwifruit, peeled and sliced

1 small Granny Smith apple, peeled,
   cored, and sliced

2 tablespoons sugar

1 tablespoon lemon juice (fresh
   or bottled)

10 to 12 ice cubes

Combine honeydew, kiwifruit, apple, sugar, and lemon juice and purée until smooth. Add ice cubes and blend until smooth and creamy. This recipe makes multiple servings; drink only one at this time.

• THE STRAWBERRY SIMPLETON •

TOTAL TIME: 5 MINUTES

SERVINGS: 4

UNDER 200 CALORIES

3 cups frozen strawberries

1½ cups low-fat milk or unsweetened
  soy or almond milk

⅓ cup strawberry jam

2 teaspoons flaxseed oil
  (optional)

Combine all ingredients in a blender and purée until smooth. This recipe makes multiple servings; drink only one at this time.

• SMOOTH TROPICAL BREEZE •

TOTAL TIME: 5 MINUTES

SERVINGS: 2

UNDER 200 CALORIES

1 cup diced frozen mango

1 cup pineapple juice

¼ cup lime juice

1 teaspoon freshly grated lime zest

12 ice cubes

Combine all ingredients in a blender and purée until smooth. This recipe makes multiple servings; drink only one at this time.

• CRAZY BANANA KIWI •

TOTAL TIME: 5 MINUTES

SERVINGS: 2

UNDER 200 CALORIES

1 medium banana, peeled and cut into
slices

1 cup low-fat yogurt

1 kiwifruit, peeled and sliced

1 teaspoon sugar or honey (optional)

8 ice cubes

Combine all ingredients in a blender and purée until smooth. This recipe makes multiple servings; drink only one at this time.

• THE BLUEBERRY ENERGIZER •

TOTAL TIME: 5 MINUTES

SERVINGS: 1

UNDER 200 CALORIES

1 cup fresh or frozen blueberries

3 tablespoons fat-free vanilla yogurt

⅔ cup low-fat milk or unsweetened
   soy milk

1 tablespoon flaxseed oil

6 ice cubes

Combine all ingredients in a blender and purée until smooth and creamy.

• THE HEARTY BANANA •

TOTAL TIME: 5 MINUTES

SERVINGS: I

UNDER 200 CALORIES

½ small, very ripe banana

½ cup fat-free plain yogurt

2 tablespoons unsalted peanut butter

⅓ cup fat-free milk

1 teaspoon honey

6 ice cubes

Combine all ingredients in a blender and purée until smooth and creamy.

• THE BOSTON GREEN MONSTER •

TOTAL TIME: 10 MINUTES

SERVINGS: 3

UNDER 200 CALORIES

1 cup chopped kale

1 medium cucumber, peeled,
seeded, and sliced

1 large green apple, peeled, cored,
and sliced

1 teaspoon fresh grated ginger

1½ tablespoons fresh lemon juice

2 tablespoons sugar

10 ice cubes

Place all ingredients except the ice cubes in a blender and purée
for 1 minute. Add the ice cubes and purée until smooth and creamy.
This recipe makes multiple servings; drink only one at this time.

• BLUE CITRUS TWIST •

TOTAL TIME: 5 MINUTES

SERVINGS: 2

UNDER 200 CALORIES

2 cups fresh or frozen blueberries

1 cup orange juice (not from
   concentrate)

½ cup fat-free vanilla yogurt

1 tablespoon flaxseed oil

8 ice cubes

Combine all ingredients in a blender and purée until smooth and creamy. This recipe makes multiple servings; drink only one at this time.

• CHEERFUL CHIPPER CHERRY •

TOTAL TIME: 5 MINUTES

SERVINGS: 4

UNDER 200 CALORIES

1 cup fresh or frozen cherries, pitted, stems removed

½ cup chopped kale

1 cup low-fat or fat-free milk or unsweetened soy milk

2 tablespoons freshly squeezed lemon juice

1½ cups water

1 teaspoon vanilla extract

1 tablespoon sugar

Combine all ingredients in a blender and purée until smooth. This recipe makes multiple servings; drink only one at this time.

• THE SWEET GEORGIA PEACH •

TOTAL TIME: 5 MINUTES

SERVINGS: 2

UNDER 200 CALORIES

2 large peaches, pitted and sliced

2 cups fresh or frozen strawberries

4 tablespoons fat-free plain or
  vanilla yogurt

6 ice cubes

2 teaspoons honey (optional)

Combine all ingredients in a blender and purée until smooth. This recipe makes multiple servings; drink only one at this time.

• BERRY APPLE SMOOTHIE •

TOTAL TIME: 5 MINUTES

SERVINGS: 1

UNDER 200 CALORIES

1 medium apple, peeled, cored, and sliced

½ cup fresh or frozen blueberries

3 tablespoons fat-free vanilla yogurt

⅓ cup low-fat or fat-free milk or unsweetened soy milk

6 ice cubes

Combine all ingredients in a blender and purée until smooth and creamy.

• SWEET BEET DETOX •

1 medium uncooked beet, chopped
   (leave skin on)

1 cup fresh or frozen blueberries

1 cup water

½ cup fat-free milk

1 tablespoon honey

1 teaspoon flaxseed oil

10 ice cubes

Combine all ingredients in a powerful blender and purée until smooth and creamy. Thin with additional water or thicken with more ice, if desired. This recipe makes multiple servings; drink only one at this time.

• THE SUNSET •

TOTAL TIME: 5 MINUTES

SERVINGS: 1

UNDER 200 CALORIES

½ cup orange juice

¼ cup pineapple juice or ½ cup
  chopped pineapple

½ medium banana, chopped

3 ice cubes

Combine all ingredients in a blender and purée until smooth and creamy.

• BLACK AND BLUE SMOOTHIE •

TOTAL TIME: 5 MINUTES

SERVINGS: 2

UNDER 200 CALORIES

½ cup low-fat or fat-free milk or
   unsweetened soy or almond milk
¾ cup low-fat plain or vanilla yogurt

1 small banana
1 cup frozen blueberries
1 cup frozen blackberries

Combine all ingredients in a blender and purée until smooth. This recipe makes multiple servings; drink only one at this time.

• AVOCADO SUPREME •

¼ cup sliced avocado

2 teaspoons lime juice

¾ cup sliced mango

1 teaspoon honey

1 teaspoon fresh mint

1½ cups crushed ice

Combine all ingredients in a blender and purée until smooth. This recipe makes multiple servings; drink only one at this time.

• THE BLUEBERRY SWIZZLE •

TOTAL TIME: 5 MINUTES

SERVINGS: 3

UNDER 200 CALORIES

2 cups fresh or frozen blueberries

6 ounces fat-free plain or vanilla
  yogurt

½ cup apple juice (not from
  concentrate)

1 medium ripe banana, peeled
  and sliced

2 teaspoons honey

8 ice cubes

Combine all ingredients in a blender and purée until smooth. This recipe makes multiple servings; drink only one at this time.

• FRUIT EXTRAVAGANZA •

TOTAL TIME: 5 MINUTES

SERVINGS: 2

UNDER 200 CALORIES

1 large banana, peeled and sliced

⅓ cup fresh or frozen strawberries

¼ cup fresh or frozen blackberries

⅓ cup fresh or frozen blueberries

½ cup fat-free plain or vanilla yogurt

½ cup grape juice or pomegranate
  juice (not from concentrate)

¾ cup low-fat or fat-free milk or
  unsweetened soy or almond milk

½ cup crushed ice, if you use fresh
  fruit instead of frozen

Combine all ingredients in a blender and purée until smooth. This recipe makes multiple servings; drink only one at this time.

• THE CHIPPER •

TOTAL TIME: 5 MINUTES

SERVINGS: 1

UNDER 200 CALORIES

2 small oranges, peeled, chopped, and seeded

¼ cup pineapple orange juice

2 small scoops orange sherbet

⅔ cup crushed ice

Combine all ingredients in a blender and purée until smooth and creamy.

• THE ORANGE BANANA •

TOTAL TIME: 5 MINUTES

SERVINGS: 2

UNDER 200 CALORIES

1 large banana, peeled and sliced

½ cup fat-free plain yogurt

1 cup orange juice

2 teaspoons honey

½ cup crushed ice

Combine all ingredients in a blender and purée until smooth. This recipe makes multiple servings; drink only one at this time.

• SWEET ANTIOXIDANT DELIGHT •

⅔ cup lemonade or 1 tablespoon lemonade and ½ cup sparkling water, chilled

⅔ cup frozen strawberries

1 teaspoon honey

⅓ cup fat-free vanilla yogurt

Combine all ingredients in a blender and purée until smooth and creamy.

• BLUE MANGO MADNESS •

TOTAL TIME: 5 MINUTES

SERVINGS: 2

UNDER 200 CALORIES

½ cup sliced mango

½ cup blueberries

½ cup fat-free plain or vanilla yogurt

1 small banana, peeled and sliced

¼ cup fat-free milk

½ teaspoon honey (optional)

Combine all ingredients in a blender and purée until smooth. This recipe makes multiple servings; drink only one at this time.

• BANANA OATMEAL BREAKFAST •

TOTAL TIME: 5 MINUTES

SERVINGS: 1

UNDER 200 CALORIES

⅓ cup fat-free plain or vanilla yogurt

⅓ cup cooked oatmeal

⅓ cup low-fat or fat-free milk or
   unsweetened soy or almond milk

¼ banana, peeled and sliced

½ teaspoon honey

½ cup crushed ice

Combine all ingredients in a blender and purée until smooth.

• THE SWEET KALICIOUS DETOX •

TOTAL TIME: 7 MINUTES

SERVINGS: 2

UNDER 200 CALORIES

2 large kale leaves, stems removed

1 small apple, peeled, cored, and
    sliced

1 cup strawberries

½ cup blueberries

¾ cup frozen strawberries
    and blueberries

1 banana, peeled and sliced

½ cup low-fat or fat-free milk or
    unsweetened soy or almond milk

½ cup apple juice (not from
    concentrate)

½ cup orange juice (not from
    concentrate)

Combine all ingredients in a blender and purée until smooth. This recipe makes multiple servings; drink only one at this time.

• CARIBBEAN GREEN POWER •

TOTAL TIME: 7 MINUTES

SERVINGS: 2

UNDER 200 CALORIES

1 cup chopped kale

1 cup spinach

½ medium Gala apple

1½ tablespoons fresh lemon juice

¾ cup water

1 teaspoon ground ginger

7 pieces frozen pineapple chunks

Dash of cayenne pepper

Combine all ingredients in a blender and purée until smooth. This recipe makes multiple servings; drink only one at this time.

• THE PLUM DELIGHT •

TOTAL TIME: 7 MINUTES

SERVINGS: I

UNDER 200 CALORIES

2 very ripe plums, peeled and pitted

⅔ cup blueberries

2 tablespoons fat-free yogurt

2 teaspoons sugar

½ cup crushed ice

Combine all ingredients in a blender and purée until smooth.

• GOLDBUG'S PURPLE MASH •

TOTAL TIME: 7 MINUTES

SERVINGS: 2

UNDER 200 CALORIES

½ cup fresh or frozen blueberries

½ cup frozen grapes

1 cup cherries, pitted, stems removed

¼ cup fat-free plain or vanilla yogurt

1 small banana, peeled and sliced

½ cup apple juice (not from concentrate)

½ tablespoon honey

½ cup crushed ice

Combine all ingredients in a blender and purée until smooth. This recipe makes multiple servings; drink only one at this time.

• THE MIGHTY GREEN POWER •

TOTAL TIME: 7 MINUTES

SERVINGS: 2

UNDER 200 CALORIES

2 cups spinach

1 medium Gala apple, peeled, cored, and sliced

2 slices cucumber, ½ inch thick

1 small banana, peeled and sliced

5 frozen strawberries

4 chunks of pineapple, fresh or frozen

1 kiwifruit, peeled and cut into chunks

1 cup coconut water

Combine all ingredients in a blender and purée until smooth. This recipe makes multiple servings; drink only one at this time.

• THE GREEN ENERGIZER •

TOTAL TIME: 7 MINUTES

SERVINGS: 2

UNDER 200 CALORIES

1½ cups kale

1 cup orange slices

1 small frozen banana

1 cup coconut water

1 cup green grapes, frozen

5 pineapple chunks

½ medium pear

¼ medium Granny Smith apple

1 pinch cayenne pepper

Combine all ingredients in a blender and purée until smooth. This recipe makes multiple servings; drink only one at this time.

[CHAPTER 9]

SUPER SHRED Soups

This chapter contains simple, inexpensive recipes that can be made in 30 minutes or less in most cases. Feel free to substitute ingredients, but be mindful of the calorie counts. You can always subtract ingredients, as that will take away calories rather than add them. You can also make modifications based on medical conditions you might have, such as allergies or high blood pressure.

In most of the recipes a serving is typically a cup unless otherwise specified. The most a serving size will be is 1½ cups. These recipes make multiple servings, so remember that you should be eating only one serving at a time. Whatever is beyond a serving either share with others or store for later consumption. These soups are meant to be fun, tasty, and healthy, so feel free to experiment with the ingredients, but do so in a smart, calorie-conscious manner. *Buon appetito!*

• WHITE BEAN AND CARROT SOUP •

TOTAL TIME: 30 MINUTES

SERVINGS: 6

UNDER 200 CALORIES

3 teaspoons olive oil

2 cloves garlic, minced

1½ (15-ounce) cans cannellini beans,
  rinsed and drained

3 carrots, peeled and sliced thin

2 leeks, white and pale green parts
  only, cleaned well and cut crosswise
  into semicircles

Two 14-ounce cans low-sodium
  chicken broth

2 cups water

2 teaspoons fresh lemon juice

1 teaspoon ground sage

Salt and pepper

Heat the oil over medium heat in a large saucepan or pot. Add the garlic and cook, stirring frequently, for a few minutes. Stir in beans, carrots, leeks, broth, water, and lemon juice and cook until heated through, about 5 minutes. Stir in the sage and continue cooking until aromatic. Season with salt and pepper to taste. To thicken the soup, mash some of the beans.

• BEAN PROTEIN EXTRAVAGANZA •

TOTAL TIME: 20 MINUTES

SERVINGS: 4

UNDER 150 CALORIES

2 teaspoons olive oil

2 cloves garlic, peeled and crushed

1 small red onion, peeled and chopped

1 cup tomato paste

1 teaspoon dried thyme

1⅓ cups fresh green beans, cut into
    1-inch pieces

One 15-ounce can cannellini beans

One 15-ounce can black beans

½ cup sliced celery

½ cup peeled and thinly sliced carrots

Salt and pepper

Heat the olive oil in a large saucepan and sauté the garlic and onion until tender. Add the tomato paste and thyme. Bring to a boil, then add all the beans, celery, and carrots. Cover and cook on low heat for about 15 minutes or until vegetables are tender. Season with salt and pepper to taste.

• SLIMMING ASPARAGUS SOUP •

TOTAL TIME: 40 MINUTES

SERVINGS: 4

UNDER 200 CALORIES

1½ pounds fresh asparagus

One 14-ounce can low-sodium

   chicken stock

½ cup water

2 yellow-fleshed potatoes, peeled and

   cut into ½-inch cubes

½ teaspoon dried thyme

2 tablespoons butter

½ cup minced leeks, whites only,

   rinsed well

½ cup minced shallots

½ tablespoon minced garlic

¼ teaspoon salt

¼ teaspoon ground white pepper

2 ounces sliced prosciutto, chopped

Trim the woody stems from the asparagus and set aside. Cut asparagus stalks into ½-inch pieces.

In a large saucepan or pot, bring stock, water, potatoes, thyme, and woody stems to a boil over high heat. Reduce heat to low, cover, and simmer until the potatoes are tender. Remove stems.

In a small stockpot, melt the butter, then add leeks and shallots and cook until tender. Add the garlic and cook until golden and fragrant. Add the chopped asparagus stalks, salt, and pepper, and cook for 4 minutes, stirring frequently. Once tender, add to the large saucepan and cover. Simmer until the asparagus is very tender, approximately 20 minutes. Remove from heat.

Meanwhile, cook the prosciutto in a small skillet over medium heat, stirring frequently until crisp, about 5 to 7 minutes.

Pour the soup into a large blender or food processor and purée until smooth. Serve the soup topped with the crisped prosciutto.

• CHICKEN AND RICE •

TOTAL TIME: 30 MINUTES

SERVINGS: 8

UNDER 150 CALORIES

8 cups low-sodium chicken broth

3 celery ribs, sliced

1 small onion, peeled and chopped

⅓ cup fresh lemon juice

Salt and pepper

1 cup long-grain rice

2½ cups cooked chicken chunks
(2 medium skinless chicken breasts)

In a medium saucepan, combine the broth, celery, onion, lemon juice, salt, and pepper; bring to a boil. Add the rice. Cook on high for 3 minutes, then reduce heat, cover, and simmer for 15 to 20 minutes. Add the chicken and let it warm through. Season with more salt and pepper to taste.

• CORN AND SQUASH SOUP •

TOTAL TIME: 30 MINUTES

SERVINGS: 4

UNDER 200 CALORIES

1 cup chopped onion

1 tablespoon extra-virgin olive oil

4 medium summer squash, diced

One 14-ounce can low-sodium chicken
   or vegetable broth

1 teaspoon lemon juice

1½ teaspoons dried thyme

1½ teaspoons dried oregano

¼ teaspoon salt

¼ teaspoon ground black pepper

3 cups fresh corn kernels
   (about 5 ears)

¼ cup feta cheese, crumbled (optional)

Heat the onion in oil over medium heat in a large saucepan or pot and sauté until tender. Add the squash, broth, lemon juice, thyme, oregano, salt, and pepper, stirring occasionally until the squash starts to soften, 5 minutes. Transfer to a blender and purée until creamy. Return the puréed mixture to the pan and stir in the corn. Bring to a simmer over medium heat, stirring occasionally until the corn is tender, 5 minutes more. Garnish with feta cheese if desired.

• CURRIED LENTIL SOUP •

TOTAL TIME: 30 MINUTES

SERVINGS: 2

UNDER 200 CALORIES

1½ cups lentils, picked over, rinsed, and drained

1 tablespoon olive oil

3 cups low-fat chicken broth

1 clove garlic, peeled and minced

1 teaspoon curry powder

1 large onion, peeled and finely chopped

1 tablespoon finely chopped celery

Combine all ingredients in a medium-size pot or saucepan, bring to a boil, then reduce to low heat, cover, and cook for 30 minutes or until lentils soften.

• TRISTÉ'S NEW CHICKEN NOODLE •

TOTAL TIME: 30 MINUTES

SERVINGS: 4

UNDER 200 CALORIES

1 tablespoon butter

½ cup chopped onion

½ cup chopped celery

½ cup chopped spinach

1 cup peas

½ cup fresh corn kernels

½ cup peeled and chopped carrots

1 sweet potato, peeled and cubed

1½ cups diced, cooked chicken meat

6 cups low-sodium chicken broth

1½ cups vegetable broth

½ cup water

½ teaspoon dried basil

½ teaspoon dried oregano

1 teaspoon poultry seasoning

Salt and pepper

1½ cups wide egg noodles

Melt the butter in a large saucepan or pot. Cook the onion and celery in butter until tender. Be certain not to overcook. Add the spinach, peas, corn, carrots, sweet potato, chicken, chicken broth, vegetable broth, water, basil, oregano, poultry seasoning, salt, and pepper. Bring to a boil, then reduce heat and let simmer until vegetables are soft. Add the egg noodles and let simmer until noodles are tender, about 15 minutes.

• CAULIFLOWER AND POTATO SOUP •

TOTAL TIME: 30 MINUTES

SERVINGS: 4

UNDER 200 CALORIES

2 teaspoons olive oil

⅓ cup finely chopped shallots

Two 14-ounce cans low-sodium
  chicken broth

3½ cups sliced cauliflower florets

4 cups diced Yukon gold potatoes

⅓ cup finely chopped celery

½ teaspoon salt

¼ teaspoon ground white pepper

1 teaspoon lemon juice

1 cup low-fat or fat-free milk

In a large saucepan or pot add oil and sauté shallots until tender.
Add the broth, cauliflower, potatoes, celery, salt, and pepper, and
bring to a boil. Reduce heat, cover, and simmer 15 to 20 minutes,
or until the vegetables are tender. Add the lemon juice. Place soup
in a food processor or blender along with the milk and purée until
smooth. Add more salt and pepper to taste.

• CHILLED CUCUMBER SOUP •

TOTAL TIME: 20 MINUTES

SERVINGS: 6

UNDER 200 CALORIES

3 cucumbers, halved, peeled, seeds scraped out with a spoon, and diced

1 teaspoon salt

5 scallions, chopped

¼ cup fresh lemon juice

2 cups low-fat buttermilk

2 cups low-fat Greek yogurt

2 tablespoons chopped fresh dill

½ cup low-sodium vegetable broth

½ cup chopped fresh parsley

Sprinkle cucumbers with salt and let stand for 15 minutes. Put cucumbers, scallions, lemon juice, buttermilk, yogurt, dill, broth, and parsley in a blender or food processor and purée until smooth. Add more salt to taste. Refrigerate for 45 minutes before serving.

• LIP-LICKING TOMATO BASIL SOUP •

TOTAL TIME: 40 MINUTES

SERVINGS: 4

UNDER 200 CALORIES

---

3 teaspoons olive oil

2 large carrots, peeled and diced

1 medium red onion, peeled and sliced

¼ cup chopped fresh basil

One 28-ounce can crushed tomatoes

One 14-ounce can chicken broth

½ cup light cream

Salt and pepper

Heat the olive oil in a large saucepan or pot over medium heat. Add the carrots and onion and cook until they start to soften, about 10 minutes. Add the basil and cook until the vegetables are tender, about 5 minutes more. Add the tomatoes and chicken broth and bring to a boil, then let simmer for 20 minutes. Allow soup to cool for 5 minutes and transfer to a blender or food processor. Purée until smooth. Return to saucepan and add the cream, stirring it in slowly over low heat. Season with salt and pepper to taste.

• BUTTERNUT SQUASH AND APPLE SOUP •

TOTAL TIME: 25 MINUTES

SERVINGS: 8

UNDER 200 CALORIES

2 tablespoons unsalted butter

1 red onion or other sweet onion,
   peeled and chopped

1 large clove garlic, peeled and
   smashed

⅛ teaspoon ground nutmeg

1 cup cubed, peeled apple
   (Fuji or Gala)

2 pounds butternut squash, peeled and
   cubed

3 cups low-sodium chicken stock

1 teaspoon ground cumin

¼ cup fat-free evaporated milk

Salt and pepper

In a large saucepan or pot, melt the butter over medium heat and add the onion and garlic. Sauté until soft, about 5 minutes. Sprinkle the nutmeg on the apples and add to the saucepan. Stir constantly for 2 minutes. Add the squash, stock, and cumin, and bring to a boil. Reduce heat and let simmer until the squash is tender. Transfer to a food processor or blender, add the evaporated milk, and purée until smooth. Return to saucepan and let simmer on very low heat for 5 minutes. Add salt and pepper to taste.

• CHICKEN CORN SOUP •

TOTAL TIME: 30 MINUTES

SERVINGS: 8

UNDER 200 CALORIES

3 cups corn (fresh or canned)

1 large onion, peeled and diced

5 cups low-sodium chicken broth

1 cup water

½ cup diced celery

2 cups cooked skinless chicken breast,
  cubed

Salt and pepper

In a large pot or saucepan, combine the corn, onion, broth, water, and celery. Bring to a boil, then lower heat and simmer for 15 minutes. Put mixture in a blender or food processor and purée until smooth. Return to pot and add in the chicken. Cover and let simmer for 10 minutes. Add salt and pepper to taste.

• STURDY SPINACH SOUP •

TOTAL TIME: 40 MINUTES

SERVINGS: 4

UNDER 200 CALORIES

½ medium onion, peeled and finely
  chopped

2 cloves garlic, peeled and minced

1 teaspoon olive oil

2 cups low-sodium vegetable or
  chicken broth

1 cup water

1 cup jasmine rice

1 stalk celery, finely chopped

One 6-ounce bag baby spinach

1½ cups low-fat or fat-free milk

Salt and pepper

In a large pot or saucepan, sauté the onion and garlic in olive oil over medium heat, 5 to 7 minutes. Add the chicken broth, water, rice, and celery to the garlic and onion. Bring to a boil, cover, and simmer for 10 minutes. Stir in the spinach, reduce heat, cover and simmer until leaves are nice and tender, 5 minutes. Reduce heat and add the milk. Let simmer for 3 to 5 minutes. Transfer to a blender or food processor and purée until creamy. Add salt and pepper to taste.

• BLACK BEAN AND TOMATO SOUP •

TOTAL TIME: 30 MINUTES

SERVINGS: 6

UNDER 200 CALORIES

1 medium onion, peeled and diced

1 tablespoon olive oil

One 15-ounce can kidney beans

One 15-ounce can black beans

2 medium tomatoes, diced

1 green bell pepper, diced

½ teaspoon garlic powder

1 cup low-sodium chicken stock

3 cups water

3 tablespoons fresh lemon juice

In a small pot or saucepan, sauté the onion in olive oil until tender, 5 to 7 minutes. Combine the onion with other ingredients in a large pot. Cover and cook on medium heat for 10 minutes, stirring occasionally, then reduce heat and simmer for 10 minutes.

• EYE-OPENING CARROT SOUP •

TOTAL TIME: 40 MINUTES

SERVINGS: 4

UNDER 200 CALORIES

2 tablespoons sweet butter

1 large onion, peeled and chopped

1 clove garlic, peeled and crushed

2½ cups peeled and diced carrots

½ teaspoon grated fresh gingerroot

2 cups low-sodium vegetable or
chicken broth

1 cup water

4 large strips of orange peel

2 tablespoons chopped fresh dill

½ cup buttermilk

Salt and pepper

¼ cup sour cream

Melt the butter in a medium saucepan. Add the onion and garlic and sauté on medium heat until tender, about 5 to 7 minutes. Add the carrots, ginger, broth, water, strips of orange peel, and dill, then bring to a boil. Reduce heat, cover, and simmer until the carrots are tender, about 20 minutes.

Remove the orange strips and transfer soup to a food processor or blender. Add the buttermilk. Purée until smooth and creamy.

Return the soup to the saucepan and add the cream, stirring over high heat until hot, but not boiling.

Add salt and pepper to taste. Top with sour cream. Serve hot.

• STUPENDOUS SWEET POTATO SOUP •

TOTAL TIME: 60 MINUTES

SERVINGS: 6

UNDER 200 CALORIES

3 medium sweet potatoes, peeled and quartered

1 tablespoon olive oil

1 medium leek, white part only, cleaned, trimmed, chopped

1 small yellow onion, peeled and chopped

½ celery stalk, chopped

1 medium carrot, peeled and chopped

1 clove garlic, peeled and minced

5 cups low-sodium chicken stock

½ cup low-fat buttermilk

Salt and pepper

Place the sweet potatoes in a large pot and cover with water. Bring to a boil, then reduce heat to medium and simmer until soft, about 15 minutes. Let cool. Meanwhile, heat the oil in a large pot over medium heat. Add the leeks, onion, celery, carrots, and garlic. Stir often until vegetables begin to soften, 5 to 7 minutes. Add the stock and sweet potatoes to the pot and bring to a boil. Reduce heat to medium and simmer until vegetables are completely soft, about 20 minutes. Transfer everything to a blender or food processor and purée until smooth. Return to the pot, stir in the buttermilk, season with salt and pepper to taste, and barely simmer over very low heat.

• BROCCOLI CHEDDAR SOUP •

TOTAL TIME: 45 MINUTES

SERVINGS: 8

UNDER 200 CALORIES

1 tablespoon butter or extra-virgin olive oil

1 medium onion, peeled and chopped

1 stalk celery, chopped

2 cloves garlic, peeled and chopped

1 teaspoon chopped fresh thyme or parsley

4 cups low-sodium chicken or vegetable broth

2 cups water

8 cups chopped broccoli (stems and florets from about 1 large bunch)

½ cup milk or light cream

1 cup cheddar cheese, shredded

Salt and pepper

Melt the butter or heat the oil in a large pot or saucepan over medium heat. Add the onion and celery and sauté until tender, about 5 minutes. Add the garlic and thyme or parsley; cook, stirring, until fragrant, about 1 minute. Add the broth, water, and broccoli, bring to a broil, reduce heat, cover, and simmer, 25 minutes. Pour soup into a food processor or blender and purée until smooth. Return soup to saucepan under low heat, add the milk or light cream and cheese. Stir occasionally while barely simmering on very low heat. Add salt and pepper to taste.

• YUMMY CABBAGE SOUP •

TOTAL TIME: 45 MINUTES

SERVINGS: 6

UNDER 200 CALORIES

1 medium onion, peeled and minced

½ tablespoon butter

3 tablespoons olive oil, divided

One 14-ounce can diced tomatoes

2 cups water

2 cups low-sodium vegetable broth

½ tablespoon instant beef bouillon

½ teaspoon garlic powder

⅔ cup carrots, peeled and diced

1½ cups celery, diced

½ green pepper, stemmed, seeded, and chopped

½ teaspoon Italian seasoning

½ teaspoon chopped fresh parsley

3½ cups chopped green cabbage

Sauté the onion in butter and 2 tablespoons of the olive oil in a medium saucepan or pot over medium heat, until softened, about 5 minutes. Combine tomatoes, water, broth, onion, beef bouillon, garlic powder, and the remaining olive oil in a large pot. Bring to a boil and simmer for 15 minutes. Add the carrots, celery, green pepper, Italian seasoning, and parsley. Simmer until vegetables are soft, about 15 minutes. Add the cabbage and simmer until tender.

In life it's always important to be able to step back, look at the landscape, and enjoy the view. You have come to the end of a sometimes challenging and significant journey. Enjoy your success and the knowledge that you have it within you to work hard, SHRED, and succeed!

Index

blueberries
    in smoothies, 176, 177, 183, 186,
        189, 190, 192, 194, 195, 199, 201,
        203, 204
    in snacks, 159, 160, 165, 168
Blueberry Energizer Smoothie, 183
Blueberry Swizzle Smoothie, 194
blue cheese, in snacks, 161, 168
Blue Citrus Twist Smoothie, 186
Blue Mango Madness Smoothie, 199
body shaping, 90–91
Boston Green Monster Smoothie, 185
bread crumbs, in snacks, 161
breadsticks, in snacks, 163
breakfast, grocery list for, 19, 58–59,
        92, 123
Breyers ice cream, in snacks, 168
broccoli
    in snacks, 162
    in soup, 224
Broccoli Cheddar Soup, 224
brown rice, in snacks, 160, 168
burritos, in snacks, 169
butter, 26
    in snacks, 160, 162
    in soup, 210, 214, 218, 222, 224, 225
buttermilk, in soup, 216, 222, 223
Butternut Squash and Apple Soup,
        218

cabbage, in soup, 225
cake spread, in snacks, 160
calorie disruption, 6–7
calories
    consumed vs. expended, 5
    food sources of, 5
cannellini beans, in soup, 208, 209
cantaloupe, in snacks, 162
carbohydrate count, 171
carbohydrates, energy from, 5
cardiovascular exercise, 14
    list of exercises, 30
Caribbean Green Power Smoothie,
        202
carrots
    in snacks, 160, 162, 166, 168
    in soup, 208, 209, 214, 217, 222, 225
cashews, in snacks, 164, 166

cauliflower, in snacks, 168
Cauliflower and Potato Soup, 215
cayenne pepper, in smoothies, 202,
        206
celery
    in snacks, 160, 165
    in soup, 209, 211, 213, 214, 215, 219,
        220, 223, 224, 225
cereal
    hot, serving sizes, 26
    in snacks, 167
cheddar cheese
    in snacks, 163, 169
    in soup, 224
Cheerful Chipper Cherry Smoothie,
        187
Cheerios, in snacks, 166
cheese, in snacks, 164, 169
cherries
    in smoothies, 177, 187, 204
    in snacks, 163, 164, 166
chicken
    in snacks, 167
    in soup, 211, 214, 219
Chicken and Rice Soup, 211
chicken broth, in soup, 208, 211, 212,
        213, 214, 215, 217, 219, 220, 222,
        224
Chicken Corn Soup, 219
chicken stock, in soup, 210, 218, 221,
        223
chickpeas, in snacks, 160, 165
chili powder, in snacks, 169
Chilled Cucumber Soup, 216
Chipper Smoothie, 196
chocolate
    in smoothies, 175
    in snacks, 161, 162, 166, 167, 168
Chocolate Razzy Smoothie, 175
cinnamon, in snacks, 160, 161, 165
Citrus-Berry salad, 159
clams, in snacks, 164
clothing sizes, drop in, with the plan,
        2, 91
cocktail sauce, in snacks, 164
coconut water, in smoothies, 205,
        206
cod, in snacks, 161

medications, and weight loss, 4
Mediterranean salad, in snacks, 165
metabolism, stoking, with snacks, 158
Mighty Green Power Smoothie, 205
milk
in smoothies, 175, 178, 180, 183,
184, 187, 189, 190, 192, 195, 199,
200, 201
in snacks, 169
in soup, 215, 218, 220, 224
mint, in smoothies, 174, 193
mozzarella cheese, in snacks, 161, 166
muffin, in snacks, 165
mussels, in snacks, 163
mustard, in snacks, 161, 167, 168

nectarines, in snacks, 163, 166
negative energy balance, 4–5
Nestlé Crunch ice-cream bar, in
snacks, 168
"no added sugar" packaging, 25,
170
"not from concentrate" packaging,
25
nutmeg, in soup, 218
nutrient density, 7–9

oat cereal, in snacks, 164
oatmeal
in smoothies, 200
in snacks, 165, 166
olive oil
in snacks, 160, 163
in soup, 208, 209, 212, 213, 215,
217, 220, 221, 223, 224, 225
olives, in snacks, 162, 166, 168
omnivorous diet, 7–8
onions
in snacks, 162, 165
in soup, 209, 211, 212, 213, 214, 217,
218, 219, 220, 221, 222, 223, 224,
225
Orange Banana Smoothie, 197
orange juice
in smoothies, 177, 186, 191, 196,
197, 201
in snacks, 159
orange peel, in soup, 222

oranges
in smoothies, 178, 196, 206
in snacks, 167
oregano, in soup, 212, 214
oysters, in snacks, 163

papayas, in snacks, 169
parfait, in snacks, 168
parmesan cheese, in snacks, 161, 165,
169
parsley, in soup, 216, 224, 225
peaches
in smoothies, 188
in snacks, 163
peanut butter
in smoothies, 184
in snacks, 160, 161, 163, 165, 168,
169
peanuts, in snacks, 162, 164
pears
in smoothies, 173, 206
in snacks, 169
peas, in soup, 214
pecans, in snacks, 164, 166
pepper
in snacks, 166, 167
in soup, 208, 209, 210, 211, 212,
214, 215, 217, 218, 219, 220, 222,
223, 224
Pepperidge Farm Goldfish, 163, 167
pickles, in snacks, 166
pineapple juice, in smoothies, 181,
191, 196
pineapples
in smoothies, 176, 177, 191, 202,
205, 206
in snacks, 160, 162, 164, 166
pistachios, in snacks, 166, 167
pita chips, in snacks, 167
plant-based diet, 7–9
Plum Delight Smoothie, 203
plums, in smoothies, 203
pomegranate juice, in smoothies,
195
pomegranates, in snacks, 163
popcorn, in snacks, 162, 163, 165
poppy seeds, in snacks, 163
Popsicles, in snacks, 168